◼ CONTENTS

■ ACKNOWLEDGMENTS

This book could not have been written without the support and encouragement of Adela de la Torre and my colleagues in the Department of Chicana and Chicano Studies at UC Davis, my academic home for the past twenty-three years. My appreciation to Angie Chabram, Miroslava Chávez Garcia, Carlos Francisco Jackson, Sergio de la Mora, Natalia Deeb-Sossa, and Maceo Montoya, whose commitment to interdisciplinarity and social justice nurtures my soul. To my *colegas y hermanas* (colleagues and sisters) Beatriz Pesquera and Ines Hernandez-Avila, who have walked along the academic path with me and were always there to watch my back. To the teachers and professors who inspired me throughout the years, Grace Chacón de Jaikel, Olene McCrary, Dave Caloca, Amado Padilla, Lonnie Snowden, James C. Coyne, and my mentors in graduate school and beyond, most particularly Ricardo Muñoz, Guillermo Bernal, and Carmen Carrillo.

To the *comadres* who inspired, supported and filled in so that I could write—Regina Armas, Lesleigh Franklin, Rosa Granadillo-Schwentker, Ellen Lanzone, Marisol Reyna Duarte, Vilma Wilcoxen, and Susan Wilde—and the *compadres* who continue to throw light on the path—Ricardo Carrillo, Sebastian Espinola, Marcelo Esteban, Samuel Tabachnik, and Hector Rivera-Lopez—your clinical skills, solidarity, and resilience have nurtured and inspired me. You constitute my *familia* of choice.

I am indebted to the hundreds of students and psychotherapy clients who taught me most of what I know. You have demonstrated that the spirit can be wounded but never destroyed. I hope that I have honored your stories and experiences in this book.

There are many people who have touched my life, among them Rebecca Carrillo, Cristiana Arruda (RIP), Christian Brother, Camilo Chavez, and Margaret Santos; your stories, conversations, and time shared challenged my thinking and strengthened my commitment. W. Ladson Hinton and Enriqueta Valdez Curiel, your solidarity and research partnerships have enriched my intellect and academic and personal life. Yolanda Martins, Emilia Moreno, Gibran Guido, Monica Siañez, Elizabeth Covarrubias, Rosa Manzo, Oscar Ureño, Marta Flores, and Rosa Velia Gomez-Camacho, the new generation of scholars who will carry on the good fight, you give me hope.

I have been able to put on paper what I have learned over thirty years of clinical practice thanks to the love and support of my family, my son Alejandro, my daughter Xochitl and my son-in-law Tyron, and their daughters, Lei-Lahni Xitlali and Naturelle Idolly Henninger. My *nietas* (granddaughters) try to keep me in balance by reminding me that I have been at the computer too long and it is time to give them attention. Their unconditional love, sweetness, inquisitiveness, and spirit keep me going during rough and calm times.

I am equally indebted to the two women and two men who were and have been my healers for most of my adult years, Carlos Stahlman (QEPD/RIP), who guided my integration of the past into a healthier present; Michelle Ritterman, psychotherapist extraordinaire, who kept me on the path of health; Camilo Chavez, who showed me that mestizo and western approaches can be used together for healing; and Ratka Mira Popovich, who helped me integrate mind, body, and spirit. You have been the guardians of my *mente, alma, y corazón*.

To the staff in Chicana/o Studies who keep me sane in times of great insanity: Alyssa West, Leticia Quintana, Kathy Hayden, and Alma Martinez. To the staff of the Center for Transnational Health at UC Davis, Linda Whent, Elizabeth Mitloehner, and Erin Weiss, your wit, support, and patience have made my life manageable. Kristen Buckles and the University of Arizona editorial staff, thank you for your understanding and support. The reviewers of the manuscript, whose careful reading and important suggestions have enriched the book, I am deeply grateful to you. Briza Perez, former student, research assistant, and reliable friend, your close attention to detail and the *Chicago Manual of Style* have made this book possible. *A todas y todos quedo eternamente agradecida;* I am forever grateful to you.

Chicana and Chicano

Mental Health

Introduction

Mental health is to be in balance; an alignment of body, mind and spirit.[1]

According to Mexican traditional healers, or *curandera/os,* health is a state of balance between body and mind, mind and heart, and body, mind, and spirit; moreover, "the health of the soul and spirit [is] at the basis of many physical and emotional ailments" (Avila and Parker 2000, 169). Health is viewed holistically and depends on the individual, family, and community being in balance with one another and with the environment and spirit world. The primary threats to health—physical, emotional, spiritual, and psychological—are rooted in imbalance. Threats to health include any and all factors that produce disharmony.

Within this belief system or explanatory model, illness is explained as deriving from social, spiritual, and physical forces (Lopez-Rangel 1996). Inherent in traditional Mexican health beliefs is the need to maintain psychological, spiritual, and interpersonal homeostasis, or balance; thus, disconnection or imbalance between soul and heart, mind and body, body and spirit is considered to be the root of interpersonal, intrapersonal, and spiritual concerns. Contemporary Mexican Americans' perceptions of health and illness—including mental health problems—often reflect a dual belief system in western or biomedical health care and "informal, complementary or parallel" care derived from traditional Mexican indigenous practices and spiritual beliefs (23).

Therefore, to facilitate the healing process of these ailments, mental health practitioners must understand the beliefs regarding the interconnectedness of the mind, body, and spirit held by indigenous Mexicans prior to the conquest, since these beliefs are also common, to varying degrees, among contemporary Mexicans and Mexican Americans or Chicana/os.[2] Furthermore, to understand and heal from spiritual, emotional, and physical distress, it is crucial to understand the sources of pain, including historical trauma brought about by the conquest and colonization of the Americas and the marginalization of Mexican Americans in the United States (Carrillo and Zarza 2008; Tello 2008).

In contrast to indigenous notions of health and illness, contemporary psychiatric and psychological explanations focus primarily on the biological basis of mental disorders. While "behavioral health" problems such as anxiety, depression, and substance abuse are understood to be influenced by both biological and psychosocial processes, preferred treatment methods, commonly referred to as *best practices,* privilege biomedical interventions (use of psychotropic medication for anxiety and depression or use of short-term cognitive behavior therapy, for example). These approaches to mental health care often neglect or minimize the historical, cultural, and social context of psychological and emotional distress and marginalize the explanatory model of affected individuals (see Bernal and Domenech Rodriguez 2012; Kleinman 1988).

■ Overview of Mental Health Care Issues

The 2010 census determined that the Latino population of the United States, that is, those persons whose cultural and historical origins are from Mexico, Central, and South America, is 50.5 million people, constituting a 40 percent growth since the 2000 census. Latinos constitute the second-largest ethnic group in the country and 16.3 percent of the US population. The largest subgroup (66 percent) is composed of Americans of Mexican descent (US Census Bureau 2011). However, it is estimated that by 2050 the Latino population in the United States will nearly double to 26 percent (Alegria et al. 2007). Mexican Americans, or Chicanos, along with Native Americans are the oldest inhabitants of the western United States. As Rios-Ellis (2005) has noted, Mexican Americans are both the oldest Latino group in the United States and also the newest arrivals. The ongoing cultural exchange between immigrants and long-term residents, as well as the proximity to Mexico and binational as well as multigenerational households, is believed to influence retention of traditional cultural practices, including health beliefs.

In the premier volume of this series, de la Torre and Estrada (2001) outlined the major factors impacting health care access for Mexicans and Mexican Americans. These include a number of important group characteristics that must be considered in the delivery of services to this population, including nativity (national origin), linguistic ability (monolingualism, bilingualism), educational attainment, occupational status, migration status (citizen, legal resident, temporary worker with permit, undocumented immigrant, refugee), and degree of familiarity with health care systems. De la Torre and Estrada also highlighted important structural or systemic barriers to health care access, among these availability of health insurance, cost of services, availability (location and hours of service), and culturally competent service providers. All these factors have equal relevance in understanding barriers to mental health care access faced by Mexican Americans/Chicanos.[3] Latinos, including Mexican Americans or Chicanos, underutilize mental health services. Among Latinos with a mental disorder, fewer than one in eleven contact mental health specialists, and fewer than one in five contact general health care providers. Among immigrants utilization rates are even lower; fewer than one in twenty use mental health services and fewer than one in ten seek such services from general health care providers.[4] A number of scholars have demonstrated that the low utilization rate by Latinos is accounted for in part by providers' lack of cultural attunement to the health beliefs of clients or patients, as well as a lack of culturally relevant services (Aguirre-Molina, Borrell, Muñoz-Laboy, and Vega 2010; Aguilar-Gaxiola et al. 2002; Alderete et al. 2000; Alegria et al. 2010; Vega et al. 1998; Vega, Kolody, and Aguilar-Gaxiola 2001).

Furthermore, in the past decade the importance of cultural competence in health care delivery has been amply documented (de la Torre and Estrada 2001; US Dept. of Health and Human Services 2001). Likewise, understanding of and sensitivity to the patient's health beliefs and illness experience have emerged as important aspects of positive treatment outcomes (Chabram-Dernersesian and de la Torre 2008; Kleinman 1988). Furthermore, in the past decade the impact of historical trauma has become the focus of attention among mental health researchers and providers. The impact of conquest and colonization on indigenous or aboriginal communities is now known to constitute risk factors for emotional and psychological distress as well as to contribute to health disparities for the generations that follow (McCubbin and Marsella 2009).

Intergenerational trauma *and* the prevalence of racism, discrimination, and institutionalized systems of oppression that emerged from conquest and domination adversely affect the spiritual, emotional, and physical well-being of Latinos and Chicanos (Duran and Duran 1995). Microaggressions, defined by Sue, Capodilupo, and associates in 2007 as the "brief and commonplace daily verbal, behavioral and environmental indignities,

whether intentional or unintentional, that communicate hostile, deroga-
tory, or negative racial, gender, sexual-orientation, and religious slights
to the targeted person or group" produce stress and affect the emotional
well-being of individuals and groups (cited in Sue 2010, 5). Microaggressions have a pernicious effect on the psyche of individuals partly because
those who perpetrate them often deny their intention to offend or blame
the aggrieved as being too sensitive or thin-skinned. Therefore, in addition
to experiencing the aggression, the targeted person's reactions and feelings are devalued, which, as Hardy and Laszloffy (2005) have noted, can
contribute to feelings of outrage, rage, and sorrow.

■ Chicano Explanatory Models

In terms of mental health service delivery, understanding the patient's or
client's beliefs regarding causality and the potential stigma associated with
a diagnosis of mental disorder are critical aspects of competent care. How
an individual explains his or her distress contributes to the type of help she
or he will seek, if any. In the 1970s, Chicano researcher Frank Newton
(1978) found that Mexican immigrants who resided in the central coastal
regions of California classified their "mental health problems" in three
ways—*nervios, locura,* and *problemas de la vida.* If the individual perceived
a nervous condition to be a result of physical illness, a physician would be
sought. If the cause was spiritual or supernatural, either a priest or a curandera would be consulted. Locura, madness or being crazy, typically was
associated with genetics and viewed as a hereditary, incurable condition or
as the result of a hex. The hex could be cured by prayer and consultation
with a specialist (curandera); the illness might be treated by western practitioners but required long-term family care and protection as well. Life's
problems were to be tolerated, faced, or worked through depending on
the nature and cause. Individuals coped with life problems through prayer
and reliance on their spiritual beliefs, through *pláticas* (conversations) with
friends or intimates, or through the distraction of work. Others expected
that time would take care of "heart" or emotional ailments. Very few consulted mental health providers.

Twenty years later, Vega and associates (1999) and Hayes-Bautista,
Schink, and Chapa (1998) found that similar explanatory models were
used by Mexican immigrants and Mexican Americans who were not highly
acculturated. In my own clinical psychology practice since 1986, Mexican

and Chicano men and women of varying socioeconomic classes and educational levels typically seek my services for problems rooted in relationship conflicts or because historical wounds (childhood abuse, early losses, and difficult family migration histories) have reopened. These spiritual, emotional, and at times physical injuries interfere with their enjoyment of life or more seriously disrupt their work and relationships with loved ones, thus causing emotional pain.

Many of my Mexican immigrant clients seek services as a result of difficulties related to their migration and the subsequent cultural adaptation challenges faced by them and their Chicana/o offspring. Rarely do these clients describe their distress using psychiatric terminology. Instead, their accounts utilize an explanatory model that often blends western and indigenous views. More acculturated Chicana/o clients may also use similar explanatory models. Ana, a twenty-six-year-old public health student, explains her distress in this way: "Sometimes I feel totally out of balance. Since my relationship ended I am not the same. I can't keep my thoughts together anymore. Sleeping is hard; she ripped out my heart when she told me she did not love me anymore. I thought we had a strong *familia* [family], but now she wants to break us up."

Ana described her distress as a state of imbalance brought about by her partner's decision to separate, breaking up the family that had been created, against all odds. Ana is a daughter of working-class immigrants and is pursuing a health career; she is excelling in her studies. She sought psychotherapy because she understood that talking to someone might help with her feelings. She was very clear that she would not take medication and therefore consulted a psychologist, instead of a physician, because she knew that her primary care doctor most likely would prescribe medication. Given her education, Ana is familiar with the mental health care system. She is an informed consumer. She has been taught that mental health problems are largely biologically based, yet she describes her distress as rooted in imbalance—her breakup has affected her heart and her mind. She sought a way to reintegrate her heart, mind, and spirit, not medication to reduce her symptoms.

Because of clients like Ana, this book offers a model rooted in mestizo psychology—the psychology of Indo-Hispanic people of the American continent—which contextualizes emotional and interpersonal ailments from both emic and etic perspectives (Ramirez 1998)[5] in order to understand more fully what ails the hearts, minds, and souls of Mexican Americans.

The case studies presented highlight the importance of understanding Chicano mental health historically and of examining the role of historical or intergenerational trauma in the experience and manifestation of emotional, psychological, and spiritual distress.[6]

Due to the cultural, linguistic, and historical diversity of Latinos, this book focuses primarily on Mexican-origin people—Chicanos—who are the largest Latino subgroup. The terms *Chicana/o* and *Mexican American* are used interchangeably throughout the book, depending on the term used by the literature cited or preferred by the individuals whose experience is being shared. Most of the mental health literature utilizes the term *Latino* or *Hispanic;* when citing studies, the term utilized by the authors will be maintained.

■ Chicana/o Mental Health: What Ails the Soul, Heart, and Mind?

Mental health is fundamental to overall health and productivity for successful contributions to family, community, and society. Throughout the lifespan, mental health is the wellspring of thinking and communication skills, learning, resilience and self-esteem.[7]

According to the Surgeon General's Report (US Dept. of Health and Human Services 2001), almost one-third of the US population has had one or more serious mental disorders. Furthermore, according to the same report, and verified by Alegria and Woo (2009), among others, individuals in the lowest strata of income, education, and occupation have higher levels of psychological distress and are more likely than those in the highest strata to have a mental disorder.

Alegria et al. (2010) propose that contextual as well as immigration and social factors play a strong role in the risk for psychiatric disorder among Latinos. Moreover, Mexican Americans and Puerto Ricans are three times more likely than European Americans to live in poverty (Caldwell, Couture, and Nowatny 2008; Williams 2005); therefore, it would be expected that the rates of psychiatric disorder would be higher. Yet their mental health *utilization* rates are lower than that of European Americans (Castañeda 2000) and most epidemiological studies find similar or lower rates of psychiatric distress among Latinos (with some exceptions that will be discussed in later chapters). This "health paradox" (higher risk and lower prevalence rates with concomitant lower service utilization) also has been found with regard to physical health (Alegria and Woo 2009; Hayes-Bautista, Schink, and Chapa 1998; Hayes-Bautista 2004).

Hayes-Bautista, Schink, and Chapa (1998), among others, have identified a number of protective factors that result in better health outcomes among Mexican immigrants, despite their more impoverished status. The same protective factors (strong family ties, healthy behaviors—less smoking and drinking—and adherence to traditional values) are used to explain the lower rates of mental disorders among Mexican immigrants. The Surgeon General's report noted that adult Mexican immigrants who have lived in the United States less than thirteen years have lower rates of mental disorders than Mexican Americans born in the United States. Similar findings were obtained in the Los Angeles Epidemiological Catchment Area Study (LA-ECA), the Hispanic Health and Nutrition Examination Survey (NHANES), and the Mexican American Prevalence and Services Survey (MAPSS) (Aguilar-Gaxiola et al. 2002), which compared rates of mental disorders among Mexican immigrants, Mexicans in Mexico City, and US-born Mexican Americans. More recently, Grant and colleagues (2004) also found that Mexican immigrants had lower rates of mental disorders than US-born Chicanos. These authors conclude that factors associated with living in the United States are related to an increased risk of mental disorders.

While the psychological literature posits that adherence to Mexican cultural values and the development of a strong ethnic identity serve as protective factors, Portes, Fernandez-Kelly, and Haller (2005) and Rumbaut (1994) note that adjustment to their new country for child immigrants and the children of immigrants depends largely on their degree of assimilation to US society. Moreover, Portes and colleagues (2005) argue that while it may be the case that most children of immigrants will eventually assimilate to the dominant US society, "it still makes a great deal of difference whether they do so by ascending into the ranks of a prosperous middle class or join in large numbers the ranks of a racialized, permanently impoverished population at the bottom of society" (1000). This process, which sociologists term "segmented assimilation," helps explain the underachievement and social problems that affect large numbers of adolescent Mexican Americans or Chicanos. These authors note that successful adaptation is influenced by a number of important factors, including the racial background of the youth and the discrimination and racism that different groups will experience, as well as the changes in the US labor market that have resulted in the rise of service employment, which is divided into menial and casual low-wage jobs and those requiring technical and professional training. While there is high demand for both types of labor, there are few opportunities in between, resulting in an "hourglass labor market," where immigrants tend to fall into the bottom, or unskilled, menial labor.

Most immigrants occupy the bottom of the labor market; their children must obtain sufficient education and develop the technical skill required to rise above the bottom of the hourglass. Such an ascent is made difficult by the poverty and crime that immigrant families often face in their communities. Portes and Zhou (1993) proposed that the adverse social circumstances many immigrants face—"the deterioration of schools, the proliferation of gangs and the occupation of the streets by the drug industry" (Portes, Fernandez-Kelly, and Haller 2005, 1009)—result in downward assimilation for their children. Such structural conditions among Chicanos have been described by Rumbaut (1994), Vigil (2002), and Barrera, Hageman, and Gonzales (2004), who argue that structural inequalities are the primary causes of Chicano youth dropping out of school and joining gangs.

While adherence to Mexican culture may provide protective factors that reduce the risk of mental disorder for a few years after immigration, the *sociocultural context* of Mexican Americans and long-term immigrants, in particular segmented assimilation, is a risk factor for emotional and psychiatric distress. Likewise, historical and contemporary trauma, as a result of colonization, marginalization, discrimination, and devaluation (Alegria et al. 2008, 2010), may contribute to psychological and emotional distress.

Historical trauma and the sequelae of racism and slavery have been documented as contributing to hypertension and other health problems as well as psychiatric distress among well-educated and high-income African Americans (Williams and Collins 1995; Williams and Mohammed 2009). Among native Hawaiians, health disparities, under-education, and overrepresentation in the juvenile and adult justice system, as well as disproportionate rates of homelessness and poverty, are accounted for by the dispossession and cultural genocide perpetrated upon them (McCubbin and Marsella 2009). These authors conclude that the physical and emotional health of marginalized individuals is adversely impacted by the burden of discrimination and racism.

Loss of language, cultural rituals, and spiritual practices creates shame and despair. The loss of culture and language often goes unmourned, because it is silenced and denied by those who occupy, conquer, or dominate. Such losses and their psychological and spiritual impact are passed down across generations, resulting in depression, disconnection, and spiritual distress in subsequent generations, which are manifestations of historical or intergenerational trauma (Duran and Duran 1995; McCubbin and Marsella 2009).

Native Americans believe that those living today are affected by what happened seven generations before. In like manner, the actions of those living today will impact their descendants for seven generations (Duran and Duran 1995; Tello 2008). Thus, contemporary Mexican Americans are impacted still by the conquest of the continent and the colonization of the southwestern United States. Their well-being and the ways in which Chicanos cope with the legacies of colonization and everyday encounters with racism will in turn influence the emotional, spiritual, and physical well-being of the next seven generations.

The emotional impact of being "othered" since childhood has been well documented (Hardy and Laszloffy 2005) as a precursor to depression, anxiety, substance abuse, and acts of aggression and violence directed toward the self and others. Acculturative stress has been linked to both psychiatric disorders and symptoms considered culturally bound[8]—*susto* (fright), *nervios* (nerves), *mal de ojo* (evil eye), and *ataque de nervios* (an attack of nerves resembling panic attack) (Guarnaccia et al. 2010; Rios-Ellis 2005).

Furthermore, the erosion or absence of cultural protective factors, along with the changes of meaning systems (cultural, social, geographic) that result from migration (Falicov 1998), as well as the erosion of community and sense of belonging resulting from efforts to acculturate or assimilate, may generate greater vulnerability to mental disorders or emotional distress among long-term Mexican immigrants and Chicana/o individuals at particular points in the life cycle. For example, Latino youth experience or engage in more anxiety-related and delinquency problem behaviors, depression, and drug use than do non-Latino white youth and are less likely to receive treatment (Castañeda 2005; Hardy and Laszloffy 2005). Mexican American girls, along with other Latinas and African American youth, demonstrate increased rates of the new morbidities—unplanned pregnancy, depression, suicidality, use of violence, and increased use of tobacco, alcohol, and other drugs (Youth Risk Behavior Surveillance System—United States 2005).

Adult Latinas, including Mexican Americans, experience double the rate of depression of men. Miranda et al. (2005) found that Latinas who immigrated to the United States without their children were 1.52 times more likely to experience depression than Latinas who immigrated with their children or who had no offspring. Mexican and Chicano men, among other Latinos, are nearly four times as likely as white non-Hispanic men to be imprisoned at some point in their lives.[9] Furthermore, those who are incarcerated are at high risk for mental disorders, compared to those who are not (Castañeda 2005).

Mexican American elderly, who will constitute a significant number of older Americans by 2050 (Hinton et al. 2006), have equal or higher rates of depression, diabetes, and dementia when compared to European Americans. Moreover, Williams (2005) found that emotional problems such as depression or anxiety impaired the daily activities of nearly one in every eight Californians aged sixty-five or older. Those most likely to report distress included people of color, those with limited English ability (particularly Mexican elders), and recipients of Medi-Cal (Hinton et al. 2006, 2008).

From a mestizo psychology model (Ramirez 1998), this book examines the explanatory models utilized by diverse groups of Mexicanos/Chicanos to describe their experience of *problemas del alma, la mente, y el corazón* (problems of the soul, mind, and heart). This is an innovative approach, as it considers both the dominant psychological paradigms utilized in the treatment of Chicanos and Latinos as well as privileges the historical, cultural, and social experiences of Mexican Americans. A central goal of the book is to situate the mental health needs and challenges of Chicanos within a historical context while responding to the contemporary realities of living in a complex, multicultural world.

The need for culturally competent mental health care providers is well established (American Psychological Association 2002; US Dept. of Health and Human Services 2001). Likewise, the barriers to mental health services encountered by Mexicans and Chicanos have been documented by many scholars, including de la Torre and Estrada (2001) and Rios-Ellis (2005). It is estimated that there are only twenty-nine Latino mental health professionals for every 100,000 Latinos in the United States, compared to 173 non-Latino white providers per 100,000 non-Latino whites. Only about 1 percent of licensed psychologists who are also members of the American Psychological Association identify themselves as Latino. It is unknown what percentage of mental health professionals can deliver services in Spanish (Castañeda 2005). Moreover, since the advent of managed care, many primary care physicians prescribe psychotropic medication, particularly anxiolytics (anxiety-reducing medications) and antidepressants, without a referral to adjunct mental health services (Hinton et al. 2006, 2007). To what extent these providers understand the cultural, historical, and emotional context of their patients' distress is unknown.

While I do not offer a review of appropriate treatment modalities to heal the hearts and minds of Chicanos, ultimately it is my hope that the information offered in this book will invite practitioners and students to go beyond best-practice models and privilege the narratives and experiences of Chicanas and Chicanos of all ages. Thus, this book is designed for both students and health care professionals who may encounter Mexican and Mexican American clients or patients in their practice.

■ Organization of the Book

Given the particular challenges and emotional issues that may affect Mexicans and Chicanos during their lifetimes, this book utilizes a life-cycle perspective to examine the psychosocial and cultural context of children, adolescents, adult men and women, and the elderly. Particular attention is paid to more vulnerable populations, that is, subgroups within the larger Chicano/Mexicano US population that may experience greater threats to their mental health: lesbian, gay, bisexual, and transgendered Mexicanos/Chicanos; children, youth, and women who experience intimate partner, family, and social violence; and the men and women whose families are torn apart by immigration policies and Department of Homeland Security (DHS) practices, including Immigration and Custom Enforcement (ICE) raids.

Utilizing a contextual and developmental approach, I explore the cultural and social factors that may contribute to mental health problems affecting Mexican Americans. I utilize a life-cycle perspective because the strengths and challenges individuals experience vary depending on their age and overall health status. This approach highlights the protective and risk factors Chicanos face in childhood, adolescence, and adulthood and thereby takes into consideration the stage of life of Chicanos and how their life experience may nuance their mental health. The first two chapters examine the ecological context of children and youth, with particular attention given to the risk and protective factors that contribute to their mental health. Available information regarding the extent of mental health problems experienced by Chicano children and youth is presented, along with cultural explanatory models.

The third chapter provides an overview of the mental health problems affecting Chicanas. I review relevant studies regarding the role of gender, culture, and class on the onset and experience of psychological distress among women. Likewise, cultural explanatory models and the subjective experience of Chicana clients are used to elucidate the biomedical and subjective experience of imbalance and psychological distress. Client narratives and women's voices are interwoven in the presentation of the most prevalent problems women experience.

The fourth chapter analyzes the role of culture, gender, class, and violence in the lives of Chicanos. The most frequent psychiatric disorders manifested among Chicanos are presented and analyzed from western and mestizo perspectives. These chapters address the complex psychosocial and cultural factors that influence the onset of mental health problems among adult Chicanos and Chicanas.

The fifth chapter examines sexuality, both as an identity and as a lived experience. The role played by cultural values and gender socialization in men's and women's experiences of coming of age as sexual beings is examined through available social-science and cultural studies, as well as the narratives of Chicanas and Chicanos.

In the sixth chapter the challenges faced by Chicana and Chicano elders are discussed, with particular attention to caregivers of elders with dementia and other chronic incapacitating diseases. Changes to the structure of Latino families as a result of migration, acculturation, and economic need often create isolation and limited resources for the elderly. As the Latino population ages, the impact on mental health created by poverty, underemployment, and marginalization throughout the lifespan must be addressed.

The conclusion offers recommendations for effective interventions, both at the level of the community and that of the family.

This book provides insights into the social, cultural, linguistic, and developmental factors that nuance the manifestation of mental health problems from childhood to old age. Two goals guided its writing: to explore the manifestation of psychological distress in this diverse population from both biomedical and cultural perspectives and to offer a context to understand the risks to the mental health of Mexican Americans in order to prevent distress and to promote balance.

■ Discussion Questions

1. How did indigenous people define mental health prior to the conquest?

2. What is meant by *intergenerational trauma*?

3. Discuss the most salient barriers to mental health care access encountered by Chicanos and Latinos.

4. What is the impact of segmented assimilation, racism, and discrimination on the mental and physical health of marginalized groups?

■ Notes

1. Student response to an in-class assignment. Course title: Chi 121: Mental Health in Chicana/o Latina/o Communities

2. The terms *Chicana/o* and *Mexican American* are used interchangeably in the text, unless quoted works or personal narratives use a different specific term.

3. Masculine nouns are sometimes used for ease of reading, and whenever appropriate, gender-specific language will be used.

4. US Department of Health and Human Services. *Mental Health: Culture, Race and Ethnicity—A Supplement to Mental Health: A Report of the Surgeon General. Executive Summary* (Rockville, MD: US Department of Health and Human Services, Substance Abuse and Mental Health Services Administration, Center for Mental Health Services), 2001.

5. *Emic* and *etic* are anthropological terms meaning, respectively, "within the group," in this case Mexicano/Chicano views on health and illness, and dominant western, biomedical views on health.

6. All names used in this book are pseudonyms.

7. US Department of Health and Human Services, *Mental Health*.

8. Acculturative stress is that derived from attempting to adjust to a new cultural context, learn a new language, and negotiate new social systems. Acculturative stress is associated with higher rates of anxiety disorder, "*nervios,*" depression, and substance abuse. See Adriana J. Umaña-Taylor and Edna C. Alfaro, "Acculturative Stress and Adaptation," in Villaruel et al., eds. *Handbook of US Latino Psychology: Developmental and Community-Based Perspectives* (Thousand Oaks, CA: Sage Publications, 2009).

9. This is a category used by the US Census to designate European Americans. Hispanics are considered to be racially white; thus, *Hispanic* is used to designate their ethnic status. *White non-Hispanic* therefore refers to all members of the white race who are not of Hispanic origin.

■ Suggested Readings

Alegria, Margarita, Glorisa Canino, Patrick E. Shrout, Meghan Woo, Nahiua Duan, Doryliz Vila, Maria Torres, Chih-Nan Chen, and Xiao-Li Meng. "Prevalence of Mental Illness in Immigrant and Non-Immigrant U.S. Latino Groups." *American Journal of Psychiatry* 165, no. 3 (2008): 359–69.

Alegria, Margarita, and Meghan Woo. "Conceptual Issues in Latino Mental Health." In *Handbook of U.S. Latino Psychology: Developmental and Community-Based Perspectives,* ed. Francisco Villaruel, Gustavo Carlo, Josefina Grau, Margarita Azmitia, Natasha J. Cabrera, and Jamie T. Chahin, 15–30. Thousand Oaks, CA: Sage Publications, 2009.

Avila, Elena, and Joy Parker. *Woman Who Glows in the Dark: A Curandera Reveals Traditional Aztec Secrets of Physical and Spiritual Health*. New York: J. P. Tarcher/Putnam, 2000.

de la Torre, Adela, and Antonio Estrada. *Mexican Americans and Health: ¡Sana! ¡Sana!* Tucson: University of Arizona Press, 2001.

Duran, Eduardo, and Bonnie Duran. *Native American Postcolonial Psychology*. Albany: State University of New York Press, 1995.

Portes, Alejandro, Patricia Fernandez-Kelly, and William Haller. "Segmented Assimilation on the Ground: The New Second Generation in Early Adulthood." *Ethnic and Racial Studies* 28, no. 6 (2005): 1000–1040.

Ramirez, Manuel III. *Multiracial/Multicultural Psychology: Mestizo Perspectives in Personality and Mental Health*. Lanham, MD: Rowman and Littlefield, 1998.

Rumbaut, Ruben G. "The Crucible Within: Ethnic Identity, Self-Esteem, and Segmented Assimilation among Children of Immigrants." *International Immigration Review* 28, no. 4 (1994): 748–94.

Sue, Derald W. *Microaggressions in Everyday Life: Race, Gender, and Sexual Orientation*. New York: John Wiley and Sons, 2010.

Sue, Derald W., Christina M. Capodilupo, Gina C. Torino, Jennifer M. Bucceri, Aisha M. B. Holder, Kevin L. Nadal, and Marta Esquilin. "Racial Microaggressions in Everyday Life: Implications for Clinical Practice." *American Psychologist* 62, no. 4 (2007): 271–86.

1

The Mental Health of Chicana and Chicano Children

Nearly one-fourth of all children in the United States who are younger than eighteen years are Latino. In 2009, 18 percent of the estimated Latino population was younger than five years old (US Census Bureau 2011), and the majority of these children were Chicana/o or Mexican American. Chicana/o children constitute the majority of births in the United States. In California, more than 50 percent of the elementary school population is of Mexican descent (Gándara, Rumberger, Maxwell-Jolly, and Callahan 2003). While there has been a great deal of research regarding the educational status of Chicana/o children and adolescents and the factors that predict achievement and school disengagement (Gándara 2005a and b; Gándara et al. 2003; Gándara, Orfield, and Horn 2006; Gibson, Gándara, and Koyama 2004), far less is known about their mental health needs.

Academic success and overall well-being are impacted by emotional health; the extent to which children can overcome challenges, maximize opportunities, and face adversity will influence how well they do in school (Grau, Azmitia, and Quattlebaum 2009). Child and adolescent mental health in turn is influenced by multiple factors, including genetics, family, and social environment, in particular poverty and health disparities, and the quality of the child or youth's relationships (Aguirre-Molina and Betancourt 2010). As the US Latino population grows and the US population overall becomes increasingly brown, it is imperative that educators and health professionals understand and safeguard the mental health of Chicana/o children and youth.

This chapter examines the prevalence and incidence of mental health problems among Chicana/o children and provides an analysis of the ecological pressures that children experience, which influence their distress. Chapter 2 focuses on Chicana and Chicano youth.

■ Explanatory Models

From a biomedical perspective, the mental health problems of children emerge as a function of the interaction between genetic predispositions, often viewed as temperament, the child's home environment, and the larger sociocultural context in which the child grows.[1] From a mestizo perspective, a child's emotional and psychological well-being rests on *the balance between his or her mind, body, and spirit,* which is in turn influenced in early childhood by the love, nurturance, and parenting he or she receives within the family and, later, by societal and environmental factors.

Prior to the conquest of the Americas, children were socialized communally. The focus of parenting was on *rooting* the children to maximize their potential by fostering purity of heart and connection to Spirit or Creator (Tello 2008). The ancient Mexicans believed that a child's destiny, *destino,* the purpose or meaning in life connected to their people, was based on his or her connection to Spirit or Creator and was predetermined (Ramirez 1998). Finding one's purpose, knowing one's destiny, was the "most significant element of keeping balanced and being well rooted" (Tello 2008, 45). Thus the parents and community guided the child's quest to find and understand his or her destiny.

During the encounter and subsequent conquest, indigenous people of Mexico were disconnected from their land. Moreover, they were forbidden to speak their language and practice their religion (Castillo 1995). Those who survived the genocide carried in their spirits, bodies, and hearts the trauma of conquest and domination. They also kept in their souls and psyches the connection to the ancestors and their past. Both the legacy of trauma and the connection to traditional values were passed on to subsequent generations. Centuries later, historical or intergenerational trauma continues to pose threats to the well-being of Mexicans and Chicanas and Chicanos (Tello 2008).

However, the historical memory of and connection to ancestral culture also remains in the spirit of Mexicans and Chicanos and serves as a potential protective factor. In contemporary times many Mexican-origin people continue to believe that how a child comes to see the world, how she understands her place in the family and in society, can either strengthen or weaken her spirit (Avila and Parker 2000). A child's physical health will be influenced by her emotional health as well. Parents and other family members are the *encargados,* those ethically responsible for and charged with the responsibility to strengthen the child's spirit through their love, guidance, and nurturance.

Jerry Tello (1994; Tello et al. 1991) proposes that the *cargas y regalos*—burdens and gifts—that parents give their children are important contributors to a child's mental health (Hurtado and Gurin 2004). The regalos (gifts) include respect, dignity, confidence, love, and affection. The cargas (burdens) are the ways in which parents belittle and devalue the children in multiple ways, sometimes unintentionally—comparing the child to his or her siblings in unfavorable ways, name calling, shaming, and humiliating. Parents' history of trauma and intergenerational trauma also can adversely impact the parenting of children. Likewise, the balance of expectations, obligations, and gifts parents bestow on their children may be a key factor in the psychological adaptation of Chicano children. In visible and invisible ways, parents may burden their children with expectations that are not age-appropriate or congruent with US cultural realities (Caldera, Fitzpatrick, and Wampler 2002). If the parents do not recognize this burden, the children may experience significant stress. Their spirits may be affected; how children see their place in the world and how they think about themselves and others may become compromised; their physical and emotional health may be impacted.

The extent to which the regalos are perceived and felt by the child may be protective. Parental love and understanding of the child's context, including the teaching of indigenous or mestizo cultural values and traditions, can help mitigate the stress produced by less supportive environments, such as the school or the social context in which the child grows. According to Hurtado and Gurin (2004), regalos are crucial in the development of a positive personal identity. Given the extended nature of many Chicano families, it is also important to recognize the role of grandparents, aunts and uncles, *madrinas* and *padrinos* (godmothers and godfathers) as potential sources of support and enculturation (Cauce and Domenech Rodriguez 2002; Falicov 1998; Minuchin et al. 1967).

In sum, from both mestizo and western psychological perspectives, the mental health of Chicano children will be determined by the health of the family and the environment surrounding the child. For optimal mental health, a child needs a strong body, mind, and spirit. In the early years, it is the parents' and extended family's responsibility to nurture that balance and to teach the child the skills necessary to thrive. Later, the school becomes an important factor in the child's mental health.

◼ Chicano Children and Mental Health

In the general US population, the majority of childhood mental health problems consist of *emotional disorders* such as depression and anxiety (including anxiety related to trauma), *behavior and conduct disorders, learning disorders* (including attention deficit disorder [ADD] and attention deficit disorder with hyperactivity [ADHD]), *pervasive development disorders,* and *schizophrenia* (Canino and Alegria 2009; Cook, Carson, and Alegria 2010).

Most childhood mental health disorders become evident when the child enters school, sometimes as early as preschool (see vignette #2, below). It is the teachers who often encourage parents to report to pediatricians the attentional and behavioral problems observed in the classroom. As a result, the majority of "problems" identified by teachers are those that impact teaching and learning—conduct disorders, hyperactivity, and attentional deficits. It is less common for teachers to become concerned about children who are anxious or depressed, as these symptoms may be mistaken for inattention or disinterest.

The extent to which Latino children in the United States are affected by psychiatric disorders is unknown, as there are no psychiatric epidemiological studies of children (Canino and Alegria 2009). However, epidemiological studies conducted in the 1980s and 1990s with Puerto Rican children and youth aged four to seventeen found that nearly 50 percent of the children on the island met criteria for a mental disorder (Canino et al. 2004). However, most of these children were functioning well at home and at school (Bird et al. 1988, 1990). If moderate-to-severe impairment in functioning was included in the diagnostic criteria, the total number of cases, or the prevalence rate, fell to 17 percent. A subsequent study compared Puerto Rican children and adolescents aged nine to seventeen years of age with European American and African American children on the mainland. Bird and colleagues (1990) found that the rates of conduct disorder and antisocial behaviors were similar across the cities. Furthermore, the island sample had lower prevalence rates of conduct, oppositional disorders, and antisocial behaviors than for children in the continental United States.

These research findings suggest that many Latino children may have symptoms of mental health problems; however, if they are learning and behaving well in school and at home, teachers or parents may not detect their psychiatric distress. A more recent study (Canino et al. 2004) found ADHD and oppositional defiant disorder (ODD) to be the most prevalent mental health problems among Puerto Rican children. Furthermore, the study authors found that only 7 percent of the children who met criteria for ADHD were receiving any treatment, including medication. Moreover, while overall rates of psychiatric illness were similar to those of European American children, when impairment in functioning was included the rates were lower among the Puerto Rican children when compared to European Americans in the same age group. What specifically is causing the distress remains unknown. However, scholars argue that a great deal of childhood anxiety and depression is the result of negotiating dual cultural pressures and expectations (acculturative stress) or problems in the family (Falicov 1998; Koss-Chioino and Vargas 1999).

Bird and colleagues (1990), Koss-Chioino and Vargas (1999), and others have concluded that child mental health and functioning at school and with peers is largely dependent on family functioning. That is, family members who are affectionate, balanced, supportive, and respectful of one another tend to raise children who are well balanced as well. These children are more likely to have a positive self-appraisal, which in turn can help them negotiate challenging situations with peers and teachers.

A number of factors have been identified as increasing the risk for psychiatric disorders in children, including exposure to violence in the family, being a child of immigrant parents who have difficulty adjusting to the new cultural context or who face chronic economic stress, or having parents who misuse or abuse alcohol and other drugs (Gil and Vega 2010). Likewise, separation from parents due to migration, incarceration, removal into foster care system, or death tends to create risk factors. Furthermore, disruptive changes, such as job loss, migration, and any trauma experienced by parents and other adults in the family can create stressful circumstances for the children, increasing the risk of emotional, behavioral, or spiritual distress (Canino and Alegria 2009; Falicov 1998; Gonzalez, Fabrett, and Knight 2010).

While no large-scale epidemiological studies have focused specifically on Chicano children, the available information indicates very low rates of mental health problems among children of Mexican immigrant parents. However, Chicano children and adolescents ages ten to seventeen have been found to be at greater risk for mood and anxiety disorders when compared with European American and African American youth of the same socioeconomic background (the Houston School Study, cited in Canino and Alegria 2009). The reasons for the higher risk are not clear; however, acculturative stress and family factors are believed to contribute to anxiety and mood disorders among Chicana and Chicano children and adolescents. Less studied has been the impact of intergenerational trauma and the ways in which exposure to microaggressions and racism, sexism, and classism impacts Chicano children (Sue 2010).

In sum, Latino children who experience psychiatric disorders generally are diagnosed with behavioral (or conduct) disorders and/or attentional deficit disorder (with or without hyperactivity). Most often, the concern about a child's behavior or mental health begins with teachers.

■ Childhood Mental Health: Explanatory Models

As is the case in other cultural groups, many Chicano parents define mental health in behavioral terms—as the absence of problems. A child who listens, obeys, and is able to learn and reach developmental milestones is considered to be emotionally healthy. The home is indeed where most childhood mental health problems are first evident; however, *how* the parents explain the troublesome or worrisome behaviors of their children (their explanatory model) and their degree of exposure to and knowledge about western psychiatric and psychological definitions of childhood problems will determine whether the parents consider the behavior a mental health issue and, in turn, whether professional mental health services will be sought.

Awareness of and knowledge about western explanatory models are greatly influenced by the level of education, socioeconomic status, and acculturation level of the parents.[2] In general, immigrant parents with lower educational attainment in their country of origin, and US-born parents with limited exposure to biomedicine, tend to rely more on cultural explanations.

The explanatory model used by parents often is rooted in their cultural beliefs. Reflecting indigenous beliefs, most Latinos believe that a child's personality is shaped mostly by the family, through genetics, parenting practices, or a mix of both (Newton 1978; Ramirez 1998; Tello 2008). The parents and extended-family members ultimately are responsible for how well a child turns out. Parents are expected to "enculturate" their children, that is, to teach them how to be members of their family and their national, ethnic, racial, and religious group. "La buena educación" (literally, good education) refers to the belief that the family provides the moral foundation and the social enculturation of the child. It is the family's responsibility to form a good person (Flores 2005a; Tello 2008).

Furthermore, most Latinos also hold that the behavior and personality of children are determined by a mix of genetics and environment. Genetics may set the parameters of what type of person a child can and will become; however, it is the family that builds character in early childhood, as well as the environment later on that will either enhance or disrupt the child's genetic potential. The belief in heredity as a factor in child behavior is evident in how families identify children's traits as belonging to one or the other parent's genealogy, as reflected in such statements as, "He has his father's temper" or, "She is *nerviosa* (anxious), like all the women in her mother's family." (See vignette #1)

■ Vignette #1: "She is just a scaredy-cat—*de todo se asusta*" (everything frightens her)

I met Anita, a nine-year-old *Chicanita,* when her parents brought her and her sister for a hardship evaluation in support of their immigration proceedings. The parents described Anita and her sister as normal children, good students, and very well behaved (*niñas bien educadas*). They stated that their children had never had mental health problems. However, they noted, Anita was *muy nerviosa* (very nervous). They laughed that she was afraid of everything—of being left alone, of the dark, of spiders and dogs. They added that she would not close the bathroom door even when she should. When I asked the parents to elaborate on Anita's nervousness, her mother stated that Anita always began to text her about thirty minutes before the end of school to make sure her mother would pick her up on time. This happened every school day. If her mother was even a few minutes late, Anita would be found crying uncontrollably. Anita's mother worked the night shift, and Anita could not sleep until her mother arrived home. When I asked the parents what they thought caused Anita's nervousness, the family normalized this behavior and laughed about it, noting that all the women in Anita's mother's family *eran unas viejas nerviosas* (were nervous women). Anita's nervousness was believed to be a personality trait. When I asked Anita to describe how and what she felt when "nervous," she shyly responded and gave classic symptoms of anxiety disorder as determined by the *Diagnostic and Statistical Manual* of the American Psychiatric Association (American Psychiatric Association 2000).

From a biomedical perspective, anxiety disorders in childhood are caused by a combination of biological and psychological factors (Costello et al. 2003). According to national figures, about seven out of one hundred children may suffer from an anxiety disorder. Girls have a greater prevalence and are at most risk if there is a family history of anxiety. Undetected and untreated anxiety disorders of childhood can disrupt a child's education and social relations, and contribute to the onset of depressive disorders and other problematic behaviors in adolescence (Costello et al. 2003). Consequently, it was crucial that the parents understand the seriousness of Anita's anxiety and the possible consequences of not providing treatment and support.

Thus, I proceeded to describe to the family the characteristics and biomedical explanations of anxiety disorder. Anita's mother began to cry and express guilt that she had not understood her daughter's suffering and in fact had often made fun of her and yelled at her out of frustration. She stated that she was a terrible parent. As I explained that anxiety disorders "may tend to run in families," she began to identify her own and her mother's and aunt's symptoms. Because Anita's symptoms began in early childhood, long before her parents' notice of deportation arrived in the mail, I could establish for immigration court (Department of Homeland Security—DHS) that Anita in fact had a psychiatric disorder for which treatment was essential. She met the criteria for hardship that would allow her parents to remain in the United States (see de la Torre, Gomez-Camacho, and Alvarez 2010).

Anita had symptoms of generalized anxiety disorder, and I needed to determine whether the anxiety was related to trauma. In particular I needed to be able to rule out any form of child abuse, as it can lead to anxiety disorders in children, and I needed to discover whether the family had experienced a significant stressor prior to the onset of Anita's symptoms. Anita's mother disclosed that her father had passed away in Mexico a few years before and that she had been unable to attend the funeral, due to her undocumented status. After his passing, she had talked incessantly about his death and was overwrought from guilt because she had not seen her father for many years. Anita then disclosed that she had "seen" her grandfather in the house after his death and had become afraid. She also was afraid that her mother would die suddenly. She had never told her mother about this. The parents concluded that Anita had suffered from susto (fright) and that given the genetic predisposition for anxiety in the family, she had developed the anxiety disorder.

The parents were able to obtain legal residency in the United States and promptly sought treatment for Anita. They also became more understanding of her fears and less punitive in their response to her "nervios." They did continue to feel shame that their family had a psychiatric problem. I underscored that from a "Mexican" cultural explanation, the more the family understood Anita's fears and worked with her to learn ways to cope with the anxiety, the stronger Anita's spirit would become, which in turn would help her "make friends" with the fear and feel safer.[3] The parents were encouraged to discuss how Anita's "vision" of her grandfather was culturally congruent. In the family's belief system, grandfather had come to say goodbye, since the family had been unable to visit before his death. Anita had seen him because as the eldest granddaughter she had a special place in the family. Anita's anxiety began to wane as she understood the cultural meaning of her "symptoms," and the parents began to feel less stigmatized.

In some families greater weight is placed on parenting practices as an explanatory model. Thus, if a child does not conform to the parents' expectations, or if she or he exhibits problematic behavior, it may be assumed that the parents have failed to parent appropriately. The problematic behavior is labeled *malacrianza*, which literally means being raised badly (by adults). Such perceptions may overlook serious developmental or emotional disorders in children (see vignette #2).

■ Vignette #2: "He is just a difficult child; *no le gusta hacer caso* (he does not like to obey)"

I met Pepito, who was four years old, when his parents brought his nine-year-old sister, Joana, for an evaluation in support of their immigration proceedings. Joana was an average student; she was classified as an English language learner (ELL),[4] because Spanish was spoken at home. While she showed some academic deficits, she did not meet any *DSM-IV-TR* diagnostic criteria. To meet the standard of hardship, children need to have a psychiatric diagnosis and experience distress *unrelated* to or beyond that which they would experience in relation to the stress of their parents' impending deportation (Cervantes, Mejia, and Guerrero Mena 2010). When I told the mother that Joana did not meet the stringent criteria for hardship of the Department of Homeland Security, she asked with some hesitation if it was normal for a four-year-old not to speak. She clarified that Pepito could speak but often seemed unwilling to respond when family members spoke to him. He also wanted everything done the exact same way all the time.

I proceeded to obtain a developmental history from the mother, who indicated that he was always that way, *desde que nació;* from birth he seemed extra irritable (compared to her daughter) and difficult to soothe. When she enrolled him in Head Start, she was told that he was different from the other children. Pepito did not play with anyone and did not seem interested in social interactions. The mother was advised that he should be evaluated for mental retardation. His mother indicated that she became angry and withdrew him from school. She decided to teach Pepito at home but had found it increasingly difficult to interact with him. He was not responsive to her physical affection; in fact, he pulled away from her and others in the family. Moreover, lately he had become aggressive toward his sister and defiant toward everyone. If anything in the house changed—his toys moved to another location, for example—he would throw tantrums and fling himself against the wall. His mother worried because in the next year he would have to begin kindergarten.

I proceeded to evaluate Pepito and made a preliminary diagnosis of autism, which is a disorder of neural development characterized by impaired social interaction and communication, and by restricted and repetitive behavior. Autism is a complex developmental disorder with a wide range of disability. The prevalence of autism has increased over the past decade, with 1 in every 150 births, and almost 1 in 70 boys. While no specific cause for autism has been identified, researchers suggest that it is likely a combination of genetic factors (Centers for Disease Control and Prevention 2008b). Other researchers propose that environmental exposure to toxins during pregnancy may be a contributing factor (Woodward 2001). Pepito's mother was a farm worker who was exposed to pesticides during her pregnancy.

As Pepito's mother began to understand the severity of her son's developmental problem, she became distraught that her lack of information had resulted in her son not receiving the help he needed for over two years. She had blamed herself for his escalating behavior problems. Her husband and extended family believed that Pepito was too *chiquiado* (spoiled—literally, infantilized); so she had become stricter and more authoritarian in her parenting. However, Pepito's behavior only worsened. So his mother came to believe that he was being aggressive "like all the men in her family" and that nothing could be done about it because it was his character and maybe his *destino*.

I explained to the mother that Pepito might have a serious developmental disorder. I also referred the family to the Regional Center closest to their hometown for further assessment. After months of failed attempts to obtain a Spanish-speaking psychologist who could evaluate him, the Regional Center diagnosed Pepito with severe pervasive developmental disorder, autism spectrum, and referred him to appropriate treatment. The parents also were provided with supportive psychoeducational classes to help them cope with and support Pepito at home. I emphasized to the mother that little was known about autism in Mexican-origin children and that a lot of studies were being done to find out the causes and to improve treatment. I encouraged her to attend the classes offered to her, because having a child with severe autism was stressful; she, her husband, and Joana would need support to continue to love and care for Pepito. In time and with treatment perhaps the family could help him negotiate his destino.

As Aguirre-Molina and Betancourt (2010) have noted, Latino parents underutilize mental health services largely due to lack of health insurance and services that are perceived as lacking cultural attunement. Moreover, boys often are problematized as aggressive since early childhood; their undesirable behaviors may be punished, and their mental health needs tend to be ignored.

In both of these cases, the parents also felt responsible for their children's "behavior" problems and attempted to change their parenting practices to remedy the situation. As stated earlier, prior to the conquest of Mexico indigenous parenting practices focused on strengthening the spirit of children and rooting them to their people and community. After the conquest, parents reportedly feared their children's loss of spirit due to the massive trauma of destruction and genocide. As a result, parenting practices were compromised, altered, and at times profoundly disconnected from the nurturing values of the ancestors (Tello 2008).

Chicano parenting practices are described as mostly authoritarian or authoritative, particularly among the working class (Flores 2005a). Authoritarian parents create and enforce rules of conduct without permitting much input from the child or offering much explanation: "Do it because I say so" and "Don't do as I do, do as I say." These parenting practices typically are more rigid and enforce traditional gender roles; thus, boys are expected and allowed to be more rambunctious, active, and aggressive, whereas girls are socialized to be more docile, obedient, and attentive to the needs of others, especially elders, parents, and younger siblings. Fathers are expected to be the disciplinarians and mothers to be the nurturers, who defer to the male authority in matters of punishment. In these families, children tend to fear and respect the authority of their fathers and revere their mothers. Rigid parenting practices, particularly if coupled with few *regalos* (gifts) and *muchas cargas* (heavy burdens), can severely affect a child's sense of worth and become manifest in problematic behavior, in how they think or feel about themselves, or in their overall emotional well-being.

Authoritative parents, by contrast, are more flexible. The rules of conduct are clear but enforced with explanations as a way to teach the child to fulfill the family's behavioral expectations. While gender role socialization may tend to be traditional, there also may be greater room for flexibility as the child enters adolescence. Authoritative parenting sometimes offers more diverse and complex models of male and female behavior. Many immigrant parents perceive parenting practices in the United States as too permissive, leading to *libertinaje,* or abuse of freedom and disrespect for the family. Some authors argue that preoccupation with the safety of their children in a new and unfamiliar context leads immigrant parents to be too strict and restrictive, thus fostering distrust of others and fear in their children (Azmitia and Brown 2002; Flores 2005a), which in turn can contribute to anxiety disorder (nervios) in childhood, and rebellion in adolescence (Carrillo and Zarza 2008; Falicov 1998; Tello 2008).

The two case studies presented illustrate how the parents' understanding of their children's behavior largely determined how they responded initially. Neither family had sought professional help for their children, because they did not define or understand the problems as requiring professional intervention. Instead, they utilized cultural explanatory models and responded with parenting practices they had learned in their homes. However, once the need for professional help was explained, they sought support for their children. Both sets of parents acknowledged that the stigma associated with seeking and receiving mental health services also got in the way. They did not want to believe their children "were crazy," which they understood was the reason people were treated by mental health professionals. Clearly, educational outreach is essential to help parents differentiate between behaviors that are problematic and difficult (malacrianza) from those that require professional consultation, such as extreme fears, excessive sadness, or developmental delays. These disorders may be ameliorated by family support and also may require professional treatment. Likewise, mental health professionals need training to evaluate childhood mental health problems in culturally sensitive ways.

■ Protective and Risk Factors: The Family and the School

In instances where the parents fail to protect, nurture, and foster the psychological development of children, the risk for mental health problems increases (Falicov 1998; Madanes 1990). This is particularly evident in families where physical or sexual abuse occurs or where children are parentified—that is, where the parents rely on their children to fulfill their own emotional needs or burden the children with tasks beyond their years. Parental dysfunction due to substance abuse or personal history of trauma may compromise parenting ability, resulting in emotional, physical, or sexual exploitation of the offspring. A number of studies find that Latina girls experience higher rates of sexual abuse than European American girls (Centers for Disease Control and Prevention 2005; Mennen 1994) and that Latina girls who were sexually abused were violated at much younger ages than their European American counterparts (see Flores-Ortiz 1997a, 1999; Mennen 1994).

Neglect and physical and sexual abuse are the primary reasons children are removed from their parents. The percentage of Latino children in foster care more than doubled, from 6.7 percent of the foster care population in 1982 to 19 percent in 2006 (Casey Family Programs 2010). In most instances, the abusive parent was engaged in substance abuse. In some cases, the mother could not protect the child due to family violence. Such parental dysfunction reflects the sequelae of intergenerational trauma and continues the chain of grief and loss, as the children are removed from the home and enter the social welfare system.

Separation from family members itself is a risk factor for depression and anxiety in children (Diaz and Lieberman 2010). Many of the Latino and Chicano children in foster care reportedly had no family member able or willing to take care of them. This situation suggests a significant breakdown in traditional family relations; there were no extended-family members available, willing, or deemed fit to take care of the child. In these cases the family was no longer a protective factor for the children. Instead, it was a source of stress, suffering, and mental health problems.

Childhood sexual abuse is associated with depression, anxiety, suicidal thoughts and attempts, and academic underachievement (Flores-Ortiz 1997a, 2003). Attachment disorders as a result of separation from the mother or primary caretaker increase the risk for depression and anxiety as well (Diaz and Lieberman 2010).

From a mestizo perspective, abuse results in susto (fright). Susto requires cleansing and the forging of new, nontoxic relationships (Avila and Parker 2000). Parental absence, separation from caregivers, and living in a climate of fear caused by family violence can all affect the neurobiology of the brain due to the massive stress experienced in these situations and may contribute to the development of anxiety and depressive disorders (Ziegler 2002), resulting in children who are perceived as being *nerviosos, malcriados,* and *tristes* (anxious, ill-behaved, and sad).

In general, psychological studies and theories posit that the family can be a protective factor for children. If the family functions well, irrespective of whether both biological parents are present in the home, the children will thrive and achieve the expected developmental milestones. In the case of children of immigrant parents, the child's adjustment to the home and school culture is optimal when the parents are able to support the biculturality of their US-born or US-raised children. If the parents are not able to support their children's "Americanization" or if the parents freeze their culture of origin (Flores-Ortiz 1993b) and expect their children to grow up Mexican in the United States without adopting US culture as well,[5] the children may not be able to adapt to the school context. Furthermore, in visible and invisible ways, parents may burden their children with expectations that are not age appropriate or congruent with US cultural expectations. If the parents do not recognize this burden, the children may experience significant acculturative stress (Canino and Alegria 2009; Umaña-Taylor and Alfaro 2009). Likewise, if the school context devalues, denigrates, or in any way belittles the culture, language, and class of the student, the child will experience psychological distress (Hardy and Laszloffy 2005).

In the 1960s Minuchin and colleagues (1967) studied low-income African American and Puerto Rican families in Philadelphia and demonstrated that extended families could foster healthy psychological development in children, despite poverty and father absence, as long as the grandmother and the mother respected each other's roles and worked together in parenting the children. However, power struggles between the women, grandmothers who took over the mother's role, or mothers who abdicated that responsibility could potentiate behavioral problems in the children. Minuchin and his colleagues made an important contribution to the psychological literature, because up until that time social scientists promoted the belief (often stated as fact) that only two-parent, heterosexual families could raise healthy and well-adapted children. Furthermore, the importance of extended family has been documented by mental health professionals consistently in the past forty years (Burnette 1999; Falicov 1998; Goodman and Silverstein 2005).

As children grow and develop, they must meet developmental milestones. In infancy the primary task is to grow and acquire new skills; in early childhood the task is to master new skills and begin the gradual process of separation from the parents and the comfort of home by attending school. These tasks are facilitated by the children's cognitive development as the brain continues to grow and develop well into adolescence and young adulthood (Siegel 2012).

The extent to which experiences of racism, marginalization, and rejection occur and impact Chicano children has not been studied systematically. However, educational research does find that brown children are often stereotyped as underachievers before they even begin school and that teachers tend to have lower expectations of English language learners (ELL), bilingual, and even monolingual English-speaking Chicano children (Garcia and Gonzáles 2006).

Whether or not children and youth face discrimination, they have to acculturate to the school context. The stress of negotiating a dual cultural system—that of the home and the school—can be assuaged by parents who are bicultural or who are aware of the different behavioral expectations and discrimination their children are likely to face in school. Studies have found that if parents prepare their children for possible discrimination and help their children develop positive self-esteem, the children are able to cope better with microaggressions and the primary cultural discontinuities they face in school (Ogbu 1978; Quintana and Scull 2009; Quintana and Vera 1999). Ogbu argued that Chicano children hold a caste status in the United States—they are devalued, dehumanized, and treated as foreigners in their own homeland. The first setting outside the family where such experiences may occur is the school; negative encounters with teachers and peers can have adverse consequences for a child's education and self-esteem. Such experiences attack a child's spirit.

Esperanza, the protagonist in Sandra Cisneros's novel *House on Mango Street*, exemplifies the dilemma faced by Chicano children when they first come into contact with school; they often have to hide their "cultural self" in order to fit in. Esperanza wishes her name was Zeze, or X, or something that her teachers could pronounce: "I would like to baptize myself under a new name, a name more like the real me, the one nobody sees" (Cisneros 1984, 11).

The clash between the school and the home culture can result in experiences of erasure for the children and may be the beginning of the devaluation of a child's cultural community, leading to a diminished sense of self that can contribute to academic disengagement and behavioral and emotional problems in adolescence (Hardy and Laszloffy 2005).

In sum, a well-functioning family that prepares the children for biculturality and possible discrimination can be a strong protective factor in childhood. Parents play a key role in preparing the children to deal with the school environment by fostering self-confidence and pride in their home culture, and by being proactive in their child's education. A well-balanced child will be able to face the developmental challenges of adolescence, a stage wherein biological changes can trigger emotional, cognitive, and behavioral problems.

■ Discussion Questions

1. How can Mexican and Chicano parents and extended-family members promote the mental health of Chicano children in the face of constant devaluation and erosion of Chicano communities?

2. How can parents inoculate their children against devaluation?

3. Discuss the *cargas* and *regalos* you received as a child.

4. Recall your first day of school. What messages did you receive about your culture, language, and ethnic or racial background from the teachers and other staff? In what way did those messages affect your academic trajectory?

■ Notes

1. From a neurobiological perspective, emotions are centered in the amygdala, a nucleus of cells in the brain that interprets information received through the senses. The amygdala then sends messages to the frontal cortex, which in turn generates responses. It is in the amygdala that experiences are interpreted as threatening, sad, joyous, and so forth; in turn, a congruent emotional response is generated. The amygdala forms part of the limbic system, which is responsible for emotional regulation and memory. Research has demonstrated that stress impairs the functioning of the limbic system through the excessive release of cortisol, a neurotransmitter, which over time may lead to difficulties with emotional regulation. Impulse control problems, mood and anxiety disorders, and substance abuse are associated with an impaired limbic system. See Daniel J. Siegel, *The Developing Mind: How Relationships and the Brain Interact to Shape Who We Are* (New York: Guilford Press, 1999).

2. Acculturation is defined as the degree to which individuals incorporate the values, traditions, practices, and attitudes of another culture, when two cultures come into contact. In the case of Chicanos, the pressure to survive and thrive in a dominant European American context may lead to behavioral (including linguistic) and attitudinal acculturation. Values emerging from the culture of origin may be modified or adapted as well.

3. "Making friends with fears" is a technique utilized in narrative therapy with children. See Freeman, Epston, and Lobovitz 1997.

4. *English language learner* is a term used to describe or characterize children whose second language is English. Terms used previously include students with limited English proficiency (LEPs), students for whom English is a second language (ESLs), or second language learners (SLLs). This shift in language is believed to represent a more accurate reflection of the process of language acquisition.

5. Culture freezing refers to the development of rigid, stereotyped values and behaviors as a result of a difficult migration process in which cutoffs from family or culture of origin occur. The immigrant family attempts to re-create, in a new context, their ideal of what a Latino family is. This ideal may be based on distorted and rigid notions of Latino culture (see Flores-Ortiz 1993b).

■ Suggested Readings

Aguirre-Molina, Marilyn, and Gabriela Betancourt. "Latino Boys: The Early Years. In *Health Issues in Latino Males,* ed. Marilyn Aguirre-Molina, Luisa N. Borrell, and William Vega, 67–82. New Brunswick, NJ: Rutgers University Press, 2010.

Canino, Glorisa, and Margarita Alegria. "Understanding Psychopathology among the Adult and Child Latino Population from the United States and Puerto Rico: An Epidemiologic Perspective." In *Handbook of U.S. Latino Psychology: Developmental and Community-Based Perspectives,* ed. Francisco Villaruel, Gustavo Carlo,

Josefina M. Grau, Margarita Azmitia, Natasha J. Cabrera, and T. Jamie Chahin, 31–44. Thousand Oaks, CA: Sage Publications, 2009.

Castillo, Ana. *Massacre of the Dreamers: Essays on Xicanisma*. Albuquerque: University of New Mexico Press, 1995.

Duran, Eduardo E., and Bonnie Duran. *Native American Postcolonial Psychology*. Albany: State University of New York Press, 1995.

Flores-Ortiz, Yvette. "Re/membering the Body: Latina Testimonies of Social and Family Violence." In *Violence and the Body: Race, Gender, and the State*, ed. Arturo J. Aldama, 347–59. Bloomington: Indiana University Press, 2003.

Tello, Jerry. "El Hombre Noble Buscando Balance: The Noble Man Searching for Balance." In *Family Violence and Men of Color: Healing the Wounded Male Spirit*, 2nd ed., ed. Ricardo Carrillo and Jerry Tello, 37–60. New York: Springer, 2008.

2

Adolescent Mental Health

The most prevalent mental health problems affecting Chicano/a youth include depression, anxiety, and conduct disorders. Young Chicano males have a high risk of accidental death, as well as death by suicide or homicide (Aguirre-Molina and Betancourt 2010). Chicanas have higher rates of depression and suicidal ideation and intent than European American and African American peers. Both Chicano and Chicana youth abuse alcohol and other drugs at rates equal to or higher than their European American peers. Yet few epidemiological studies have focused exclusively on the mental health of Chicana/o youth.

The Houston School Study (cited in Canino and Alegria 2009) found that Chicano preadolescent children and adolescents ages ten through seventeen were at greater risk for mood and anxiety disorders when compared with European American and African American youth of the same socioeconomic background. The reasons for the higher risk are not clear; however, acculturative stress and family factors are believed to contribute to anxiety and mood disorders among Chicana and Chicano adolescents. The impact of intergenerational trauma and the ways in which exposure to microaggressions and racism, sexism, and classism impacts Chicana/o adolescents have not been studied.

This chapter examines the particular psychosocial needs of Chicana/o youth and the protective and risk factors associated with their mental health.

■ Identity/ies

The most important task of adolescence is to develop an identity and a sense of belonging. Hurtado and Gurin (2004) distinguish between personal and social identities. Personal identity is an aspect of the self that is composed of psychological traits and dispositions that make the individual unique. These traits are fairly stable and are formed within the family. Social identities, however, encompass the aspects of the individual's self that derive from their knowledge of membership in a particular group, such as gender, class, and ethnicity (Hurtado and Gurin 2004). Moreover, race, class, gender, sexuality, and ability at times are stigmatized. While an adolescent may identify with a particular racial, ethnic, or cultural group, she may lack the awareness that her social identity is stigmatized. Micro-aggressions and overt racism threaten the adolescent's sense of self (Hardy and Laszloffy 2005).

Likewise, in adolescence the increased influence of peers, friends, and nonfamilial relationships, including those with teachers, calls for youth to balance familial and nonfamilial relationships (Falicov 1998). For Chicano youth developmental tasks also include developing a positive identity, as well as learning to negotiate social contexts that often devalue their ethnicity and their parents' country of origin. The current backlash against Mexicans, whether documented immigrants or not, fosters a hostile social milieu. While both males and females must negotiate multiple identities in adolescence, for girls this process takes place within a larger context that often devalues their gender and is rife with gender violence (Gallegos-Castillo 2006). The personal and social identities of Chicano males often are racialized and "othered." Brown males, from the age of thirteen, are feared and viewed in stereotyped ways as gangsters or potential delinquents, irrespective of their class status and home location (Hardy and Laszloffy 2005). For Chicanos and Chicanas identity formation entails developing a sense of self that is gendered, and which negotiates ethnic and racial characteristics and sexual identification and preference, while experiencing varying degrees of marginalization (Hurtado and Gurin 2004).

Depending on the home culture, the family's socioeconomic status, and the youths' social milieu, adolescents may need to develop identification with two or more countries, value systems, languages, and ways of being. It is quite understandable that Chicana/o adolescents experience massive amounts of acculturative stress, which can potentiate the development of psychological problems (González et al. 2010; Umaña-Taylor and Alfaro 2009). The task of ethnic/racial identity formation may be even more challenging for mixed-raced Chicanos.

According to the 2010 census, Latinos are increasingly mixed-race, with parents of various Latino national origins or ancestries (Mexican and Salvadoran, for example) or parents who are European American or members of another ethnic group. In one of my studies of adolescents in the 1990s, more than half of the Latino sample were mixed, and included Mexican and Middle Eastern, Chicano and Asian, and Mexican and African American (Flores-Ortiz 1994). Several of the adolescent girls in another study identified themselves as Blaxicans (Black and Mexican [Flores 2006]). For them, an additional element of identity formation was identifying with two racial and ethnic groups, while simultaneously negotiating their place within the dominant European American culture of the school. Julieta, a fourteen-year-old high school freshman, described her experience this way: "Mom is Mexican and Dad is black. I am being raised Mexican, but I don't really fit within either group. I am too black to be Mexican and too brown to be black. So I hang out with other girls who don't fit anywhere either."

Gurin and Morrison (1980) distinguish between identification and consciousness in ethnic identity development. Awareness of stigmatization is referred to as consciousness—because it entails working to change the conditions of the group to which the youth belongs and thus improve the lives of others (Hurtado and Gurin 2004). While personal and social identities may form early in adolescence, consciousness may take longer to develop and to understand contextually. Julieta identified as "Blaxican." She had created her own ethnic label. She felt stigmatized and "othered" by both Chicano and African American peers; she tried to make the most out of it by finding a peer group that faced similar challenges.

For youth who are questioning their sexual preference or who are gay, lesbian, bisexual, or transgendered (LGBT), the identity formation process may be more complicated, given the expectation in traditional Latino families that children will grow up, marry, and produce offspring (Trujillo 1997). In addition, the degree of homophobia present in the youth's family and community will also determine how safe it is to "come out" and claim a sexual identity other than heterosexual. As Morales (1990), Espin (1999), and Rodriguez (2004) have noted, a gay or lesbian adolescent may first disclose his or her sexual orientation to a sibling, a friend, or an ally. Coming out to traditional immigrant parents is often quite difficult and fraught with anxiety and, at times, depression.

■ Vignette #3: "Please make my son heterosexual; who will carry on our family name?"

Jason, a seventeen-year-old, third-generation Chicano male, was brought to therapy by his parents in the hope that I could convince him to become heterosexual. Jason was seen by his high school counselor because the teachers were concerned by his low academic performance. Up until ninth grade he had been a model student. Of late, however, his grades had begun to drop. His English teacher was concerned that Jason might be depressed. His counselor was able to help him identify that he was very anxious and depressed as a result of coming to terms with his sexuality. He was afraid of disappointing his conservative, second-generation Christian Mexican American parents, who expected him to succeed academically, marry, and have a family. Jason's counselor had spoken to his mother but felt that a family therapist might be more effective in explaining to Jason's father that homosexuality was not an illness. After several family meetings, both parents came to understand that Jason needed their unconditional love and support to recover from depression and that their acceptance of his sexuality was crucial for his psychological well-being. While the parents continued to struggle with their belief that homosexuality was a sin, they wanted their son to be happy and healthy. They offered him their love and support; however, they demanded that Jason hide his sexuality from the extended family. Jason was referred to a gay Chicano therapist who would treat his depression and help him deal with the demands of his family and support his coming-out process.

In some of my earlier work (Flores 2006), I discussed the ethnic identification of young Chicanas and how a strong sense of belonging to a racial/cultural/ethnic group served as a protective factor, as it facilitated their decision making regarding high-risk behaviors—drinking, smoking, and premarital sex, which are among the most prevalent health problems facing adolescent Chicanas (Denner and Guzmán 2006; *State of Hispanic Girls* 1999). Moreover, many of the girls in my study experienced being stereotyped and racialized by teachers who assumed that all girls with Spanish surnames were Mexican or immigrant, while the majority were in fact US-born. Few teachers bothered to ask about their students' or their families' national origins.

Students in the ninth and tenth grades of urban high schools who participated in my study demonstrated largely a Mexican or Chicana identity that was unexamined. They used ethnic labels used by their parents or older siblings, without much consideration of what they meant (Flores 2005a). As Bernal and Knight (1993) and others have noted, from the time they are in elementary school, Chicano children will have a sense of their identity; however, the meaning of that identity may not be fully understood or explored until college or later in life, unless the parents teach and explain to their children what it means to be Mexican or Chicano.

Having cultural awareness and knowledge provides youth with a sense of belonging that can counter the noxious impact of marginalization and racism (Hurtado and Gurin 2004). From a mestizo psychology perspective, knowing one's racial, cultural, and ethnic roots is key to understanding one's destino (Ramirez 1998). Without a sense of who they are ethnically and culturally, *and* lacking acceptance by the dominant culture, youth may internalize the negative stereotypes and externalize their distress through "acting out," or behavioral problems (Hardy and Laszloffy 2005); some youth may embody the negative stereotype, while others may internalize the distress and develop anxiety or mood disorders (Koss-Chioino and Vargas 1999).

From a mestizo perspective, the lack of affirmation of the youth's multiple identities, marginalization, and microaggressions will injure the spirit and the heart of the young person. Problems of gender, sexual, and ethnic identity resulting from devaluation are often at the core of adolescent psychological distress (Hardy and Laszloffy 2005). Unless educators and family members are aware of and knowledgeable about the complex developmental tasks of youth of color, they may augment the stress experienced by the youth.

■ The Role of the Family in Adolescent Mental Health: Parenting Practices in Adolescence

Many immigrant Latino parents "tighten the reins" on their adolescent children, particularly their daughters, to ensure that they will follow *"el buen camino,"* the good path, which will lead to *"la buena vida,"* the good life (Flores 2005a; Grau, Azmitia, and Quattlebaum 2009). Immigrant and less acculturated parents often expect their children to remain connected primarily to their family and home. This expectation may create stress for youngsters, who feel pressured by the culture outside the home to become independent, move out, and become an adult, even if they feel unprepared to do so.

Parents who hold traditional values tend to be stricter in their socialization practices, to ensure that their children will follow the good path (Falicov 1998; Flores 2005a). Thus, these parents may be concerned about their children's friends and extrafamilial activities. A lot of traditional socialization is done through *dichos,* or sayings, that convey moral lessons and parental expectations—*"dime con quien andas y te dire quien eres—"* (Delgado-Gaitan 1994).[1] If the youth understands the cultural context guiding parental expectations, she or he may be able to decode indirect parental messages. In fact, studies find that many parents do not explicitly state their expectations about behavior—alcohol and drug use and sexuality, for example—with their children. When they do, girls in particular feel closer to their mothers and are able to negotiate with peers and romantic partners on matters of risky behaviors, and in turn feel more efficacious in protecting themselves (Flores 2006; Flores, Tschann, and Marin 2002; Romo et al. 2006). However, when parents are not able to guide their adolescent children, youth may seek support outside the family, in their peers or dominant culture institutions, which may or may not lead the youth to the "good path."

Parents often describe problematic adolescent behavior as *"falta de respeto"*—lack of respect. What parents at times do not specify is what exactly is not being respected—the culture of the parents, the parental expectations, or their hopes and aspirations for their child. If the parents and children have not developed good communication in childhood, it will be more difficult to establish in adolescence, when it will be critical for parents and children to understand each other (Falicov 1998; Bernal and Flores-Ortiz 1990).

■ Vignette #4: A problem of disrespect

Oliva was fourteen when her parents brought her to treatment, after she was found to be cutting school during the summer and going instead to the movies. Her parents, hardworking Mexican immigrants who had four older male children, were at a loss as to what to do. They worried that Oliva *iba en mal camino* (was on a bad path). By cutting school she was jeopardizing her academic success, which the parents viewed as essential to her future.

Oliva replied that she was doing well in school and was going to summer school *only* to get out of the house, since she was "a servant to her parents and siblings." Her parents were most offended by her depiction and complained that Oliva was increasingly disrespectful. Oliva replied that her family did not respect *her*. She had to cook for her brothers and wash and iron their clothes, on top of doing her own schoolwork and working after school to have her own money. She needed a break and that is why she went to the movies.

In the exchange between the parents and Oliva, their different cultural expectations become evident. The parents expected Oliva to fulfill traditional gender roles. Oliva considered it to be unfair. She complained that her brothers did not even thank her for all she did. The parents replied that serving her brothers was her obligation. Oliva disagreed. Oliva and her parents did not speak the same language, both figuratively and literally. Oliva preferred to speak English, and her parents Spanish. They also held different ideas about gender roles.

The parents expressed concern that by going to the movies alone, Oliva endangered not only her reputation, but also her life. The family lived in a neighborhood plagued by crime. Oliva retorted that she knew how to take care of herself, since in walking to school she encountered multiple risks—from sexual harassment to racist comments to drive-by shootings. The parents were horrified at this, since they left for work very early and were unaware of the daytime dangers their daughter faced. Oliva, in turn, began to speak more openly about the stressors she faced at school, the multiple assaults on her mind and spirit as a result of racist curricula, prejudiced teachers, oversexed boys, etc. She wanted to come home and find respite from all that; instead, she found work to be done, unrealistic expectations, and lack of understanding. She felt like exploding, she said.

The parents had planned to drop her off at my office in hopes that I could "knock some sense into her." They had come to see me, despite my being a "*locóloga*"—literally, a crazy people doctor—because their Chicano priest, a personal friend of mine, had recommended me highly as someone who understood Mexican families. However, I had insisted that the entire family should come for the first meeting so that they could help me understand what was going on with their daughter.

The family came for a few meetings where we worked on creating greater balance and fostering more justice in the family relationships *and* finding ways to increase Oliva's safety in her world. The parents began to attend school meetings and advocate for their daughter; they also were willing to place fewer housekeeping responsibilities on Oliva and instead to demand that their sons contribute to the upkeep of the home. Efforts were made to bring greater emotional closeness among the siblings and between Oliva and her mother, who had become estranged.

These suggestions were designed to help the family direct Oliva into the good path while respecting her own needs.

■ Protective Factors

Most scholars agree that the family can be the most protective factor for adolescents. However, due to the dramatic cultural changes occurring over the past twenty years, pressures from the larger social context at times overshadow the influence of the family. Luis Vargas (Koss-Chioino and Vargas 1999) offers an ecological model to understand the complexity of growing up Chicano in the United States. He proposes that the mental health of youth is supported best by a family that prepares the adolescent for adulthood by allowing increasing independence while providing a supportive and loving environment in the home. Parents who understand the challenges of negotiating multiple cultures, languages, and social demands can foster a sense of competence and efficacy in their children. Most authors agree that promoting biculturality and teaching the youngster pride in his or her culture of origin while supporting his or her biculturality is optimal to reduce acculturative stress (Gallegos-Castillo 2006; Umaña-Taylor and Alfaro 2009). Furthermore, to fully understand the complexity of the Chicano youth's experience, one must evaluate not only the role of the family but that of the peer system and the larger social system and structures with which the youth interacts, most notably the schools and, in some cases, the social welfare and juvenile systems. Knowledge about the "lifescape" (Koss-Chioino and Vargas 1999) or life space of youth (Hurtado and Gurin 2004) is critical to make sense of troubling and dangerous adolescent behavior.

Several important family protective factors can facilitate Chicanas' and Chicanos' development in adolescence, including

1. A positive relationship with the mother, particularly for girls (the role of fathers has not been studied extensively)
2. Enculturation within the family to develop a strong and positive cultural identity with concomitant knowledge of the culture of origin
3. Parental and extended family support of biculturality
4. Parental involvement with the school
5. Support for the youth's increasing independence
6. Positive communication between parents and children

7. Positive and consistent male role models for Chicano boys and young men
8. Identification with and pride in culture of origin, which provides rootedness and a sense of belonging

Carrillo and Zarza (2008) and Tello (2008) suggest that a great deal of Chicano youths' despair and problematic behavior is the result of father or male absence. Tello notes that a mother can take a male child to the bridge; however, she cannot teach him how to cross it. Thus, positive male role models and mentors are crucial for the healthy emotional and social development of Chicano males.

■ Risk Factors

As is the case with younger children, there is a dearth of epidemiological data on Chicano adolescent mental health. The Houston Study (in Canino and Alegria 2009) found that Mexican-origin youth were at greater risk for depression and anxiety. A report by the National Coalition of Hispanic Health and Human Service Organizations (*State of Hispanic Girls* 1999) described the mental health problems of young Latinas as "new morbidities." Teen pregnancy, depression, suicide attempts, anxiety, family and social violence, substance misuse and abuse, and use of weapons have been on the rise among Latina adolescents. In fact, since the late 1990s Latinas have surpassed African American girls in their rates of depression and suicidal behavior. While the rates of substance abuse have declined among US high school students, Latina adolescent substance abuse rates have increased (Ortegon and Werner 2008).

Most at risk for depression and suicide are US-born daughters of immigrant parents who have difficulty negotiating parental demands for maintaining traditional values, behaviors, and practices from the parents' home country, and who have a poor relationship with their mothers. These girls despair because they do not feel understood by their mothers and feel unable to fulfill the expectations and demands emerging from both cultures. Often the crisis erupts around issues of gender and sexuality. While the mother expects her daughter to embody traditional values of virginity and proper conduct (whether or not the mother practiced them herself), the girl's new social context may be more permissive, and new cultural practices of sexual expression and freedom may seem more appealing than traditional gender role behaviors expected in the home (Deardorff, Tschann, and Flores 2008; Ortegon and Werner 2008).

Also at risk are second-generation Chicanas who live in poor neighborhoods in urban settings and who encounter both sexism within the family and racism at school as well as increasing social violence (Gallegos-Castillo 2006). These young women at times find positive solutions to the pressures they face—stealing time away from family obligations and creating personal time to go to the movies, for example. Other times, young women comply with parental expectations and internalize their distress. Historically, adolescent and adult males have engaged primarily in externalizing behaviors, that is, aggression and high-risk actions that endanger their lives—drinking and driving, fighting, gang membership, use of drugs—reflecting depression, despair, and a profound lack of belonging or a psychological homelessness (Baptiste, Hardy, and Lewis 1997).

A concern about conduct disorder in childhood is that it may evolve into delinquent behavior; both of these are markers of adult antisocial personality disorder. This disorder in turn is associated with incarceration (Castro 2005; Poe-Yamagata and Jones 2000; Poe-Yamagata and Wardes Noya 2005). That is, incarcerated males typically have a history of conduct or oppositional defiant behavior in childhood and delinquency in adolescence.

In the past, females tended to internalize their difficulties; depression, anxiety, lack of belonging—the sequelae of trauma were experienced and suffered quietly or expressed primarily through self-injurious behaviors such as cutting, disordered eating, suicidal ideation, and suicidal behavior. Increasingly, girls externalize their distress as well (Hardy and Laszloffy 2005; *State of Hispanic Girls* 1999).

Youth aggression and violence has become a public health concern. The leading causes of death for Latino males ages fifteen to twenty-five are accidents, homicide, and suicide (Centers for Disease Control and Prevention 2008b). Hardy and Laszloffy (2005) posit that the roots of youth violence directed toward the self and others rest on experiences within the family and society. Specifically, violence on the part of adolescents, whether directed toward themselves or others, is "a reformulation of societal pressures that are grounded in the complex intersection of race, class, and gender politics" (61). The sociocultural context of a youth, in particular how the youth was socialized in the home, nuances the specific manifestations of violence. Internalized oppression and hatred of "the other," which may be a mirror of oneself, contribute to black-on-black and brown-on-brown violence.

There are four aggravating factors that contribute to youth violence—devaluation, disruption or erosion of community, dehumanization of loss, and rage (Hardy and Laszloffy 2005).

Devaluation

Experiences of marginalization, stereotyping, "othering," and being rendered invisible may result in feelings of devaluation. Devaluation may occur both within and outside the family. In some instances devaluation occurs continually, for example, when parents demean and criticize their children as a means of socialization. In other instances, situational devaluation can occur as a result of parental abuse or neglect, parental abandonment (even if only temporary or for an economic reason, as in the case of transnational migrations, including deportation). Situational devaluation also can occur as a result of divorce or peer rejection.

Societal devaluation can and often does occur in multiple and gender-specific ways for youth of color in general, through the criminalization of males as evident in the high rates of incarceration in juvenile detention facilities for transgressions that would result only in probation for European American and affluent adolescent males (Poe-Yamagata and Wardes Noya 2005). Hardy argues that youth of color *know* that they are perceived as criminals and that they are devalued because of their gender and their ethnicity or race, and sometimes class.

Both male and female adolescents encounter institutionalized racism and classism; from childhood, their language and culture is devalued; their appearance may be ridiculed, rejected, or attacked. The impact on girls emerges from attacks on the self through colorism. As one adolescent client once asked me, "Why don't they make *chola* Barbies?" She continued, "How am I supposed to feel good about myself if all I see is whiteness?" Latina and Chicana females also experience objectification—if noticed at all, they may be cast as exotic sex symbols. In adolescence fitting in and looking good are paramount. Standards of beauty that do not reflect the diversity and indigenousness of Chicanas can be a significant source of stress, in some cases contributing to disordered eating— binging, purging, and using laxatives to lose weight and appear more "Anglo" or as a means to manage stress (Chamorro and Flores-Ortiz 2000).

For poor and working-class youth, societal devaluation also may emerge through classism and class-based assumptions. The societal perception that most, if not all, Chicanos are poor, immigrant, and undocumented erases the experience of middle-class Chicana/o youth who never lived in a barrio. Such stereotyping can lead to within-group "othering," as more economically privileged Chicanos may not want to be confused with those who are stereotyped and marginalized, resulting in a denigration of less economically advantaged or educated Chicanos and a distancing from or disidentification with their ethno-cultural roots, because "you have to dress the part" (Hardy and Laszloffy 2005). Failed efforts at passing for European American in order to fit in or being rejected by other Latinos and Chicanos for being "whitewashed" may produce distress as well.

Another source of devaluation is the inherent heteronormativity and heterosexism in most cultures,[2] which silences the sexual expression of LGBT youth and attacks a core aspect of their identity. Many youth of color who are gay or uncertain about that aspect of their identity feel that there is no room to question their sexuality within traditional or highly religious families. Thus LGBT youth often suffer in silence. They may internalize the homophobia present in their families or culture and attempt to deny their sexuality. They may develop mood disorders, which can lead to suicide. The suicide rate among gay youth is four times higher than that of their heterosexual peers (Massachusetts Dept. of Elementary and Secondary Education 2007; Mustanski, Garofalo, and Emerson 2010).

Experiences of devaluation irrespective of their source and form result in soul wounds. When the essence of a person— his or her appearance, sexuality, culture, and language—are demeaned and devalued, the spirit suffers. Likewise, the hearts and minds of Chicanas and Chicanos who are marginalized and othered will suffer. Mental health problems may ensue.

The devaluation that youth experience within and outside the home often results in aggression. Men of color turn their aggression toward women and their symbolic selves, other men of color—simultaneously committing homicide and suicide (Hardy and Laszloffy 2005). Latinas and other girls of color are more likely to turn the rage against themselves—in cutting and suicidality—and, in some cases, against other girls or their own flesh and blood (*State of Hispanic Girls* 1999).

Disruption of Community

Youth violence can also be understood in terms of the disruption in their communities as a result of migration, poverty, high crime, and negative police–community interactions (see Gallegos-Castillo 2006). Hardy argues that a strong connection to community serves as a buffer against devaluation.

However, the disruption of community robs youth of a sense of security, connectedness, acceptance, and identity, which in turn may lead to loss of hope and diminished compassion and empathy for others. "To be alienated from community is to be alienated from one's humanity, and when this occurs, the potential for violence increases dramatically" (Hardy and Laszloffy 2005, 65).

Hardy and Laszloffy distinguish among three levels of community— primary, extended, and cultural communities. The primary community includes the family. Among Chicanos, family often incorporates both blood relations and fictive kin such as *padrinos* and *madrinas* (godfathers and godmothers). The extended community is constituted by the neighborhood, the school, community centers, and churches. The extended community can serve as a protective or risk factor for youth. The disruption of these communities as a result of migration, poverty, high crime, and marginalization can create experiences of devaluation for youth. *Cultural communities* refers to the youth's gender, sexuality, ethnicity, race, and class, which are critical during adolescence. Cultural communities may have intangible borders and may be invisible to parents and other adults. Youth need to feel a part of both the family and the peer system. Cultural communities serve to acquaint one with one's own intersectionality—the way in which oppression based on race, class, ethnicity, sexuality, gender, and ability interact, creating multiple and simultaneous forms of marginalization.

Youths who identify as Chicana/o and have identity consciousness are more likely to understand how social inequalities are created and serve to oppress Chicana/os as a group. Such awareness can transform the rage of injustice into social action. Without such consciousness, experiences of injustice may fuel rage.

Extended communities may be disrupted by external factors such as poverty and limited resources, natural disasters, or migrations—whether from one neighborhood or country to another—and by internal factors such as struggles for power in organizations and among peer systems. Being popular and fitting in are very important for most adolescents, and the criteria for popularity may be group specific; however, being considered an outcast or being bullied can have enormous psychological consequences for youth, including depression and suicide (Hardy and Laszloffy 2005).

Cultural communities may be disrupted by racism, sexism, classism, and homophobia. They also can be disrupted by attacks based on religious beliefs and cultural practices. The anti-immigrant, anti-Mexican policies enacted by Arizona (Arizona AB 1070) and proposed by many other states, allowing police to stop and demand documentation of anyone who "looks Mexican," attack and denigrate the sense of self, resulting in feelings of lack of acceptance and belonging among many Chicanos and other Latinos in the United States. These policies also may trigger distress resulting from earlier or historical trauma. For example, parents who fled their countries as a result of persecution or violence and came to the United States to seek protection, and to prevent their children from experiencing similar trauma, may be revictimized by discriminatory laws and policies. As parents see their children being victimized as well, a climate of despair and fear may develop in the home that will impact the youths' mental health.

Dehumanization of Loss

Chicanos historically have experienced many losses—land, resources, language, culture, and loved ones. Losses are cumulative and additive and can be traumatic, resulting in intergenerational posttraumatic stress disorder (PTSD) (Duran and Duran 1995). However, many of these losses have not been acknowledged by others. A loss that is not recognized by others, Hardy agues, becomes dehumanized—the loss of all losses. Furthermore, when a person is devalued, she or he is objectified, stripped of beinghood, and rendered invisible. Thus, the losses experienced may become invisible and unacknowledged, resulting in unmourned and unhealed losses and wounds. This may be the beginning of intergenerational trauma and a multigenerational risk factor for grief, anxiety, and depression among Chicana and Chicano youth. How can one grieve the losses caused by racism when the existence of racism is denied?

Many Chicano youth experience the loss of peers and family members to social violence, particularly in urban settings. In some communities the building of altars and streetside memorials to victims of crime occurs on a monthly basis. Many youth appear desensitized to the grief of such losses as the pain is masked by anger and rage (Hardy and Laszloffy 2005).

■ Vignette #5: "I don't care; your words can't hurt me"

Lola was fourteen when her best male friend, Eddie, was shot by young men from a neighboring town. Lola stopped going to school and ran away from home after a fight with her mother. Her mother was in shock when she heard about Eddie's death; although she had known Eddie since he was a small child, her main concern was for her daughter's safety. Without thinking about the impact of her words, she blurted out, "What kind of friends do you have that get shot at?" Her daughter ran out of the house and returned home only when the police found her after three days.

Lola was enraged. Her mother's words meant to her that Eddie's life had no value. Eddie was not worthy of grief. Eddie was not the first friend who had died. With each death, her "heart hardened." Lola said that nothing mattered any more. "Why go to school? You could be dead tomorrow."

As a member of a devalued cultural and gender group—Chicana and adolescent—Lola was accustomed to marginalization and being stereotyped. However, she had expected more understanding and compassion from her mother. Lola stated, "My mother's words broke me; they broke my heart and spirit. But it doesn't matter, I don't care, words can't hurt me anymore."

It took considerable time and work with a compassionate therapist and adolescent group for Lola to reengage with school and to find meaning in Eddie's death. Reparation of her relationship with her mother was also difficult, but her mother's continued support and accountability—admitting that she had spoken from fear and not from the heart when responding to Eddie's death—facilitated their reconciliation.

Other youth experience the loss of familial support and a concomitant loss of trust in the government as a result of the deportation of one or both parents in ICE raids. Other youth may face the untenable choice of remaining in the United States with relatives or moving to Mexico with their parents as the adults seek to adjust their status in order to reenter the United States with proper documentation. The disruption of family and community created by such situations leads to massive stress for children and youth (Cervantes, Mejia, and Guerrero Mena 2010).

Devaluation and disruption of community threaten the psychological well-being of youth because they represent losses. The dehumanization of such losses can significantly impair the mental health of youth and potentiate rage, the final factor contributing to adolescent violence.

Rage

Anger is a normal reaction to a perceived injustice; if appropriate opportunities for its expression exist and the anger is validated, it is likely to pass quickly. However, suppressed, denied, forbidden anger fuels itself and is the seed of rage—an intense, sustained, and consuming emotion. If rage is suppressed and unexpressed (due to limited opportunities for healthy expression—cultural expectations, for example, that women not show uncontrollable anger lest they be considered crazy)[3]—it grows, intensifies, and can lead to violence. Furthermore, rage may be a defense against more vulnerable emotions; it may mask the pain of multiple wounding as a result of devaluation, erosion of community, and dehumanization of loss. If males are socialized not to cry or show signs of "weakness of character," rage may become an outlet to display their grief and despair.

In the case of men of color who express rage, society further punishes them by detention, incarceration, or violent response; this in turn leads to further dehumanization of loss, devaluation, and erosion of community. Although more visible now, the incarceration of Chicano youth is nothing new (Chávez Garcia 2012).[4] As reported by Arévalo, Bécares, and Amaro (2010), in 2005 Latinos made up 20.2 percent of prisoners in federal and state correctional institutions, and 15 percent of inmates in local jails. Most of these men began their "criminal careers" as juveniles. Hardy posits that there is always a history that underpins the rage felt and expressed by youth of color, a history that must be rendered visible, acknowledged, recognized, and channeled to avoid its eruption into violence.

In a recent study of adolescents, Shetgiri and colleagues (2010) found that depression may increase the risk of fighting for Latino youth and that perceived support at school could serve as a protective factor. In their study, Latinos who said they felt supported by at least one person at their school were less likely to fight, while European American teens who perceived support from their families were also at decreased risk of violence (Shetgiri et al. 2010). These authors concluded that the key to mitigating teen violence was support from parents *and* teachers, particularly for Latino males.

Chicano children and youth must be valued in the home and inoculated against the racism, marginalization, and devaluation they are likely to experience outside the home. The erosion of Chicano communities must be countered with community action and positive outlets for youth. Educational systems must be changed and held accountable to educate and respect the youth. Schools can play a crucial role in supporting the emotional well-being of youth. Furthermore, social policies must be challenged if they devalue, denigrate, erase, or otherwise assault the bodies, minds, and spirits of Chicano children and youth.

■ Lesbian, Gay, Bisexual, Transgendered, and Queer (LGBTQ) Youth

Few studies have focused on the mental health needs of LGBTQ Chicano youth. While all of the foregoing issues apply to these youth, it is critical to consider the extent to which homophobia within the family further increases youths' experience with devaluation and erosion of community. Chicano families that can accept their children's sexual orientation can buffer the external devaluation, while families that ostracize their gay children create further losses (as was evident in Jason's family). In the general youth population, lack of familial and societal support is a risk factor for depression and suicide among gay youth (Mustanksi, Garofalo, and Emerson 2010).

In recent years bullying in schools has become a major concern. A number of high-profile suicides were reportedly related to bullying. Nationally, in recent years, children as young as eleven have committed suicide, after having endured relentless bullying at school (Friedman et al. 2006; Gould et al. 2004). The bullying often takes the form of antigay taunts and harassment, even when the children being bullied are not gay. Sexuality when used as a weapon of denigration can profoundly impact the mental health of young people. Devaluation of their sexuality results in an erosion of a youth's cultural communities, generating profound grief. As long as school administrators and educators as well as families continue to ignore the importance of supporting an adolescent's sexual identity, LGBTQ youth will continue to die, for they often feel that their death would be celebrated by those who are supposed to love them (Gould et al. 2004).

■ Summary

In sum, the most prevalent mental health problems affecting Chicano/a youth include depression, anxiety, and conduct disorders. Young Chicano males have a high risk of accidental death as well as death by suicide or homicide (Aguirre-Molina and Betancourt 2010). Chicanas have higher rates of depression, suicidal ideation, and intent than European American and African American peers. Both Chicano and Chicana youth abuse alcohol and other drugs at rates equal to, or higher than, their European American peers. Given the increase in youth violence and the disproportionate incarceration of Chicano youth, it is imperative to understand the preventive role of the family and the school. Both systems must be strengthened to provide adolescent Chicana/os with the tools to maintain or regain balance in their lives as they transition to adulthood.

■ Discussion Questions

1. How can Mexican and Chicano parents and extended-family members promote the mental health of Chicano youth in the face of constant devaluation and erosion of Chicano communities?

2. How can parents inoculate their children against devaluation?

3. Discuss the types of microaggressions you experienced in your adolescence.

4. How might you build your own resilience to withstand the multiple assaults you may face or have encountered in your lifetime?

■ Notes

1. In English, "Tell me who your friends are, and I will tell you who you are."

2. Heteronormativity is the cultural bias in favor of opposite-sex relationships of a sexual nature, and against same-sex relationships of a sexual nature. The assumption is that all people are heterosexual and abide by norms that apply to their group. As a result, lesbian and gay relationships are subject to a heteronormative bias.

3. *Ataque de nervios*, considered a culture-bound syndrome among Puerto Rican and other Latinas, is characterized by excessive emotion and rage. Women with this condition experience anxiety, uncontrollable crying, and excessive rage.

4. Historian Miroslava Chávez Garcia (2010) documents the incarceration of Chicano youth in California between the late 1800s and the mid-1900s. Chicano children as young as eight were often confined in correctional "schools" due to family problems or what today would be considered conduct disorders—disobedience and oppositionality. Undoubtedly, many of these youths were reacting to situations of injustice and were criminalized and punished in return.

■ Suggested Readings

Aguirre-Molina, Marilyn, and Gabriela Betancourt. "Latino Boys: The Early Years." In *Health Issues in Latino Males,* ed. Marilyn Aguirre-Molina, Luisa N. Borrell, and William Vega, 67–82. New Brunswick, NJ: Rutgers University Press, 2010.

Canino, Glorisa, and Margarita Alegria. "Understanding Psychopathology among the Adult and Child Latino Population from the United States and Puerto Rico: An Epidemiologic Perspective." In *Handbook of U.S. Latino Psychology: Developmental* and Community-Based Perspectives, ed. Francisco Villaruel, Gustavo Carlo, Josefina M. Grau, Margarita Azmitia, Natasha J. Cabrera, and T. Jamie Chahin, 31–44. Thousand Oaks, CA: Sage Publications, 2009.

Castillo, Ana. Massacre of the Dreamers: Essays on Xicanisma. Albuquerque: University of New Mexico Press, 1995.

Denner, Jill, and Bianca Guzman, eds. Latina Girls: Voices of Adolescent Strength in the United States. NY: New York University Press, 2006.

Duran, Eduardo E., and Bonnie Duran. Native American Postcolonial Psychology. Albany: State University of New York Press, 1995.

Hardy, Kenneth V., and Tracey A. Laszloffy. Teens Who Hurt: Clinical Interventions to Break the Cycle of Adolescent Violence. New York: Guilford Press, 2005.

Hurtado, Aida, and Patricia Gurin. Chicana/o Identity in a Changing U.S. Society: Quien Soy? Quiénes Somos? Tucson: University of Arizona Press, 2004.

Koss-Chioino, Joan D., and Luis A. Vargas. Working with Latino Youth: Culture, Development, and Context. San Francisco: Jossey-Bass, 1999.

Quintana, Stephen M., and Nicholas C. Scull. "Latino Ethnic Identity." In Villaruel et al., Handbook of U.S. Latino Psychology, 81–98. Thousand Oaks, CA: Sage Publications, 2009.

Romo, Laura F., Claudia Kouyoumdjan, Eram Nadeem, Marian Sigman. "Promoting Values of Education in Latino Mother–Adolescent Discussions about Sexuality." In Latina Girls: Voices of Adolescent Strength in the United States, ed. Jill Denner and Bianca L. Guzmán, 59–78. New York: New York University Press, 2006.

Tello, Jerry. "El Hombre Noble Buscando Balance: The Noble Man Searching for Balance." In Family Violence and Men of Color: Healing the Wounded Male Spirit, 2nd ed., ed. Ricardo Carrillo and Jerry Tello, 37–60. New York: Springer, 2008.

Velasquez, Roberto J., Leticia M. Arellano, and Brian W. McNeill. The Handbook of Chicana/o Psychology and Mental Health. Mahwah, NJ: Lawrence Erlbaum, 2004.

3

Gender and Mental Health

Depression, Anxiety, and Substance Abuse among Chicanas

In the general population, the primary mental health diagnoses affecting women are major depression and anxiety disorders—in particular posttraumatic stress disorder (PTSD) as a result of gender and sexual violence (Alegria et al. 2007; Herman 1992) and intergenerational trauma. Women are likely to experience depression at twice the rate of men (Centers for Disease Control and Prevention 2010). A number of factors are associated with women's higher rates of depression, including genetics, hormonal changes, and environmental and sociocultural context. Feminist scholars, including Jean Baker Miller (1974) and her colleagues at the Stone Center, argue that women's position in society contributes to women's higher rates of depression. This is particularly the case with women of color, who generally encounter multiple forms of gender discrimination and violence throughout their lifetimes (Alegria et al. 2007).

Epidemiological studies find that nativity is a risk for lifetime psychiatric disorder among Latinas. Living in the United States is a risk factor for depression among women of Mexican origin and Mexican immigrants. US-born women who are English-language dominant are more likely to have experienced depression, anxiety, or substance use disorder than are immigrant women. The greater risk is attributed to pressures to acculturate—acculturative stress—and the need to navigate different cultural expectations (as discussed in chapter 2), which increases the risk for emotional distress (Delgado 2002; Torres 2010). Likewise, their psychological distress may be related to segmented assimilation, which results in underemployment, limited upward mobility, and possibly greater exposure to violence if the women live in high-crime urban centers or barrios (Rumbaut 1994). The risk is higher for third-generation women than for immigrants or second-generation Chicanas. Latinas also experience higher rates of depression than Latino men and rates similar to European American women (Alegria et al. 2007).

Chicanas often attribute their emotional distress to *problemas de la vida* rooted in relational difficulties with family members—in particular parents, partners, and children. They also attribute emotional distress to role strain, economic pressures, or immigration problems faced by loved ones. Depending on their stage of life, Chicanas may focus primarily on relationships with parents, friends, intimate partners, and children, and in later years, on aging parents and grandchildren. Not prioritizing their own emotional needs tends to affect women's sense of self, their self-esteem, and their sexuality (see Flores et al. 2009).

Many adult Chicanas also experience in adulthood the sequelae of childhood parental separation, sexual and physical victimization, adult intimate partner violence (IPV), and sexual violence, which impact a woman's spirit, mind, and body. As a result of such trauma, Chicanas may experience anxiety, depression, and increased risk for substance misuse or abuse (see Flores-Ortiz 1995, 1999, 2004; Flores 2005a).

Over the past thirty years, many scholars have described the position of Latinas within the larger US society and the family and examined the role of gender discrimination and sexual violence in the mental health problems of women (Perilla, Bakeman, and Norris 1994; Ramos Lira, Koss, and Russo 1999; Ramos Lira, Saltijeral, and Saldivar 1995; Rodriguez et al. 2008, 2009; Russo and Denious 2001). These scholars conclude that irrespective of the primary cause of emotional distress, the *sociocultural context* of Latinas and the women's explanatory model of mental health must be taken into account to fully understand and respond to their psychological, spiritual, and physical complaints. This chapter provides an overview of mood, anxiety, and substance abuse disorders and how adult Chicanas experience and express their emotional and spiritual distress.

◼ Explanatory Models

From a cultural perspective, mental health problems may be caused by imbalance from or within relationships, or imbalance between the heart, mind, and body. Chicanas who utilize a traditional explanatory model may categorize emotional problems as *nervios*, which in turn can be defined as a physiological manifestation of interpersonal imbalance. The cause of nervios is related to an individual not being true to his or her word (relational), not living in integrity, or experiencing discord within important relationships. Symptoms include bouts of crying, tension, listlessness, loss of appetite, irritability, and sadness (Avila and Parker 2000; Salgado de Snyder, Diaz-Perez, and Ojeda 2000).

Mental health problems can also have spiritual causes: *mal puesto* (hex or curse) can be caused by a *brujo/a* (witch) or could be a punishment from God. Symptoms may be behavioral or reflected in negative attitudes; *tristeza,* or sad emotions, may also be symptomatic of a hex. *Envidia*—envy—also may lead to *mal de ojo* or *mal ojo* (evil eye), an illness caused by staring, coveting, or envy by someone who has a very powerful look. As a result, the recipient of mal de ojo may experience physical distress (fever, chills, general malaise, or nervios). The mestizo explanatory model holds that when someone is the object of envy, she gets sick in her *tonal* (spirit). Envy is an energy contrary to love and can be transmitted with or without intention. Trauma, including intergenerational trauma, also can lead to emotional disorders, as traumatic events affect *alma, cuerpo, mente, y corazón* (soul, body, mind, and heart) (Avila and Parker 2000).

Chicanas also may view problemas de la vida as the result of bad luck. Central to this belief is the notion that the energies and expectations we put into life have a direct effect on what happens to us. If we invest negative energy (shame, worry, fear) into things, we may face negative outcomes (Avila and Parker 2000).

The way a woman understands her distress, whether she attributes her malestar to nervios, to *locura*, or problemas de la vida, or to biomedical reasons, will influence the likelihood of her seeking any mental health services, whether traditional or professional.

■ Mood Disorders

From a western, biomedical perspective, mood is defined as the experience of emotion. While most individuals may experience temporary sadness as a result of loss, stress, or problemas de la vida, a mood disorder is characterized by a disturbance in *the experience and manifestation of mood.* To be considered a clinical syndrome, the mood disorder must last longer than two weeks and affect the individual's work, family, and social life. The *Diagnostic and Statistical Manual of Mental Disorders* (American Psychiatric Association 2000) determines the criteria for classification of eleven types of mood disorder.[1] Two of the most common mood disorders are depression and bipolar disorder. As stated, the most prevalent mental health problem among Chicanas is major depression.

Major Depression

This is the most common mood disorder among women, who are twice as likely as men to be diagnosed with the condition. It is also the most common mood disorder among Latinas. The symptoms of depression—feelings of sadness or despair that do not go away, loss of appetite, sleep disturbance, worry, anxiety, and feelings of guilt—can negatively affect a person's ability to function effectively in the activities of daily living, such as going to work and school, caring for family, and taking care of basic needs. More than 20 million people in the United States have depression, according to the National Institutes of Health (National Institute of Mental Health 2005). Prolonged and untreated major depression can result in thoughts of suicide and suicide attempts.

Risk Factors

From a biomedical perspective, depression is explained as the result of an imbalance in the brain of neurotransmitters, including serotonin, norepinephrine, and dopamine, which function within areas of the brain that regulate emotions and mood. Depression also may occur as a result of specific situations, including traumas or stressors, such as the loss of a loved one, job loss, prolonged unemployment, separation, or divorce.

Environmental factors, such as poverty, overcrowding, and exposure to social violence, may also play a role in the onset of depression. A normal reaction to an abnormal situation, such as natural disasters, may also trigger symptoms of depression or a mood disorder. Depression may run in families and may be transmitted intergenerationally in women, particularly if the family has experienced historical trauma (Priel and Besser 2002).

As discussed in chapters 1 and 2, the family is expected to provide a sense of security for children. Attachment, the type and quality of bonding between a parent (typically the mother) and her infant, can serve as a protective or risk factor for adult relationships and mental health. Separation from parents in childhood may result in ambivalent or anxious bonds, which in turn create vulnerabilities to adult depression. Maternal depression may affect how a child forms relationships later in life and may increase the risk for a daughter's depression in adulthood, particularly if no other maternal figures are available (such as a loving, kind grandparent). Current research efforts are searching for specific genes that may be involved in passing a tendency toward developing depression in family lines (Priel and Besser 2002). In sum, major depression may have both biological and social antecedents.

As discussed in chapter 2, Latino youth have a higher prevalence of depression than European American adolescents. The higher prevalence continues into adulthood for Chicanas and may well be influenced by the same risk factors—acculturative stress, difficulties balancing gender role obligations (role strain), economic pressures, and problemas de la vida that have become chronic or that overwhelm coping mechanisms. Difficulties attaining and maintaining balance in roles, obligations, and relationships are considered risk factors for depression in women (Baker Miller 1974).

Feminist scholars (Baker Miller 1974) propose that because women are socialized to be relational beings for whom *being in* a relationship is a central task of adult development, relationship challenges or problems may bring forth *problemas del corazón*—heartache—which can evolve into depression (Avila and Parker 2000). Loving too much, *empacho emocional,* can result in feelings of rage and profound disappointment when relationships do not work out, despite adherence to traditional cultural scripts. Prioritizing others over oneself, which often is expected of women in traditional cultures, contributes to major depression in women, particularly if their investment in relationships does not generate positive outcomes. Julia, a forty-five-year-old, second-generation, working-class, divorced mother of two adolescent children, was diagnosed with depression by her primary care physician a few months after her husband left her. She expressed her distress in this way: "I was sold the bill of goods—be a good wife, loyal, loving, self-sacrificing . . . and for what? He left me for someone who does not even know how to cook. Now he is the one doing the cooking . . ."

Whether the primary contributor to depression is biological or sociocultural, or a combination of factors, it is critical to understand how the woman affected by depression understands *and* experiences her distress. As described in the introduction, Ana sought therapy after her partner decided to separate. Ana complained of a pervasive sense of sadness; she had trouble focusing in school, difficulty managing her emotions, and feelings of hopelessness. While Ana was pursuing a career in the health field, her family remained most important. As she put it, "I put all my eggs in this basket—I thought we had a family—and now she is breaking us up." The loss of her familia implied a disconnection from her daughter on a daily basis and a loss of her foundation. She felt as if the ground under her feet had become unstable: "My *tapete* (rug) was removed," she stated.

For college-bound Chicanas leaving home may be a risk factor for depression, particularly if there is insufficient support from parents who fear that they will lose their daughter or that she will change too much away from their gaze and protection. Young Chicanas often experience loyalty pulls between obligation to family and a desire to pursue their own dreams. The culture shock experienced once they arrive on a college campus may also trigger depression, particularly if they encounter further devaluation and microaggressions (Stebleton et al. 2010; Sue 2010).

The developmental task of young adulthood is to solidify identity and form stable relationships; the implication for women is that they will find their soul mate and marry. For women who do not prioritize marriage, who are not heterosexual, or who do not find a suitable partner, family and social pressures and expectations to marry and have children may contribute to the onset of depression.

In some of my earlier work I documented the role of acculturation and marital stress in the onset of depression in women (Flores-Ortiz 1993a). Immigrant women who stated a preference for more egalitarian relationships showed lower rates of depression than women who conformed to traditional gender roles, although traditional women described their marriages as happier. Among Chicanas, balancing role expectations rooted in traditional values and their own more "contemporary" job or educational aspirations was a source of distress, because they were *supposed* to prioritize the needs of others over their own desires.

Across the life cycle, Chicanas are expected to fulfill familial obligations that are gendered: daughter, girlfriend/partner/spouse, sister, cousin, mother, grandmother, madrina, friend, *comadre,* etc. In her study of Chicanas along the US–Mexico border, Norma Williams (1990) found that working-class women experienced less role strain than professional women, because blue-collar workers identified primarily as mothers and wives. They worked to supplement the family income. Chicanas who had pursued an education and career identified primarily as professional and less as mother/wife. Yet they were expected to fulfill familial obligations. Consequently, they experienced more role strain and less marital satisfaction, as did the professional women in my study (Flores-Ortiz 1993a).

Elena Flores and colleagues (2004) examined marital conflict and acculturation among Chicano husbands and wives. Their findings demonstrate that with increased acculturation, both men and women are more likely to express their conflicts openly and directly. At times, bicultural husbands experience their wives as more physically and verbally aggressive, which potentially can disrupt the marriage and contribute to emotional distress in both partners.

In sum, depression is a disorder with multiple causes. Thus, it is critical to examine and understand women's social, cultural, and political positions in society and how gender, acculturation, and acculturative stress, as well as social class, shape women's lives across the life cycle (see Moraga and Anzaldúa 1983).

Bipolar Disorders

Mood disorders also include manic episodes, mixed episodes, bipolar 1 and 2, and premenstrual dysphoric disorder. Their prevalence is about 1 percent of the population. Men and women are equally likely to be affected. Manic episodes are characterized by symptoms such as increased self-esteem, increased motor activity, and pressured speech, which may be troublesome to the family but not to the affected person. Often there is a reduced need for sleep, increased talkativeness, or flight of ideas or racing thoughts, and the person is easily distractible. Poor judgment (spending sprees, sexual adventures, and foolish investments) is also characteristic of a manic episode. In severe cases, a manic episode may include psychotic features, a disconnection from reality, which requires hospitalization to protect the individual and others. Bipolar disorder often entails impairment in work, social, or personal functioning. The individual experiencing a manic episode is often euphoric and expansive; she or he also may have irritability. To meet criteria according to the *DSM-IV-TR,* the duration must be of at least one week, and the disorder must not be caused by substance abuse, in particular, amphetamines or cocaine, which often leads to manic-like behaviors.

Bipolar 1 (previously known as manic-depressive illness) is a cyclic disorder that includes at least one manic episode among individuals who have experienced depression. Men and women are equally affected, for a total of about 1 percent of the general population. There is a strong hereditary component. The disorder is defined by the occurrence of *spontaneous* depression, manias, and hypomanias (elevated mood without some of the more serious symptoms of a manic episode).

When Latinas experience bipolar 1 disorder, they may be perceived by their families as suffering from locura, particularly if they engage in sexually inappropriate behavior. If family members are not familiar with the symptoms of this psychiatric disorder or have only limited information about its symptoms, the affected woman may be viewed as promiscuous, irresponsible, or crazy. If the symptoms begin to manifest in young adulthood, the parents may view the behavior as characteristic of the libertinaje rampant in the United States. The family may become punitive and restrictive and not seek treatment.

Bipolar 2 entails a lesser degree of disability and discomfort than bipolar 1. This disorder consists of recurrent major depressive episodes interspersed with hypomanic episodes. Women may be more prone than men to develop bipolar 2; however, because it is relatively rare, with less than 1 percent prevalence in the general population, it may not be diagnosed accurately or result in appropriate mental health treatment, particularly if the family or the Chicana herself fears stigmatization.

As stated, Chicanos may view mania and bipolar disorder as locura or as symptoms of ataque de nervios (Lewis-Fernandez et al. 2002). In the Latino explanatory model, locura is a severe form of chronic psychosis, which includes incoherence, agitation, auditory and visual hallucinations, inability to follow rules of social interaction, unpredictability, and possible violence. An individual experiencing a manic episode may experience *celajes*—seeing shadows—which must be differentiated from visual hallucinations that are symptomatic of schizophrenia and other psychotic disorders. As a result of the symptoms, the family and friends of the affected woman may view her as "unstable, irritable, or difficult." The family may not recognize that she is experiencing a psychiatric disorder. Luis, the husband of Lupe, a forty-two-year-old Chicana diagnosed with bipolar 2 disorder by a psychiatrist, explained his wife's symptoms this way: "She has always been *corajuda* (ill-tempered). With the change (perimenopause), she has gotten worse. One day she is happy or content, the next she is screaming at me and at the kids. We are at our wit's end. Her chronic spending has me in the poorhouse. I think she went crazy."

Lupe, however, believed that Luis was cheating on her and that his lover had hexed her. She was insistent that her husband's lover had made her sick due to envy. Luis was adamant that he was faithful and that no other woman existed. He viewed his wife's beliefs as proof of her locura. In this case, Luis actually was relieved to learn that his wife had a psychiatric disorder that often produced delusions or false beliefs, and that the disorder could be treated.

After she was diagnosed and the family was referred to family therapy with me, the couple's children and Luis became more understanding and compassionate and rallied to help Lupe agree to take medication to manage the symptoms. While Lupe was unconvinced of her husband's fidelity, she agreed to try medication to feel less depressed. She agreed to do it because her children begged her to try medication. Thus, she did it for them, not for Luis or even herself. However, she insisted on obtaining a *limpia,* or cleansing, from a local curandera to remove the hex. The family supported her and accompanied her to obtain a family cleansing, as their relationships needed to be rebalanced as well, given the disruptive nature of Lupe's symptoms and how they as a family had reacted to the symptoms.

Thus, from a cultural perspective, mood disorders can be understood as rooted in relational imbalance or as the result of hexes, envy, or trauma, or as symptoms of locura.

■ Anxiety Disorders

The *DSM-IV-TR* identifies several types of anxiety disorder, including panic disorder, agoraphobia without history of panic, specific phobia, social phobia, obsessive-compulsive disorder, post-traumatic stress disorder (PTSD), acute stress disorder, generalized anxiety disorder (GAD) and anxiety disorder due to a general medical condition.

There is a strong genetic component to anxiety disorders; they tend to run in families and may first become evident in childhood (as discussed in chapter 1). Anxiety disorders can also occur as a result of a stressful life event and, in the case of PTSD, as a result of traumatic or life-threatening events.

Anxiety disorders are often viewed as nervios by less-acculturated Chicanas and as resulting from role strain or relational difficulties (problemas de la vida). They can also be caused by mal de ojo, hexes, or trauma, or can be viewed as a character trait (*ser nerviosa*), rather than as a psychiatric disorder (Avila and Parker 2000).

Panic Disorder

Panic disorder is a common anxiety disorder found in as much as 3 percent of the general adult population (compared to 10 percent for panic attack in general). It is especially common among women, and typically symptoms first appear in young adulthood. The disorder is diagnosed when, after an attack is experienced, the individual's worries about having another one interfere with activities of daily living, such as driving to work or being in crowded places. As a result, the affected person will do just about anything to avoid a panic attack; thus, he or she may avoid driving or going to locations similar to or reminiscent of the location where the attack occurred.

Panic Attacks

Panic attacks can be quite incapacitating, leading to life changes—avoiding places or situations similar to those where the first attack occurred (e.g., airports, malls, or while driving), which in turn can result in becoming reclusive or developing specific phobias (fear of heights, of driving, or of leaving the home). Panic attacks can occur as isolated experiences in young adults or as part of other anxiety disorders, medical conditions, or substance abuse disorders. Onset is generally in the twenties, and the lifetime prevalence is about 10 percent of the general population.

During a panic attack, the individual suddenly develops a severe fear or discomfort that peaks within ten minutes. During the attack common symptoms include chest pain or other chest discomfort, chills or hot flashes, a choking sensation, derealization (feeling unreal), or depersonalization (feeling detached from oneself). The affected individual may also feel dizzy, lightheaded, faint or unsteady; nausea or other abdominal discomfort may occur, as well as numbness or tingling, sweating, shortness of breath or a smothering sensation, and trembling. As a result of the symptoms, those affected believe they are having a heart attack or some other *physical* health problem. When the person believes she is having a heart attack because of the chest pains, she is more likely to seek medical attention. Therefore, most referrals to mental health providers due to panic attack are the result of emergency room visits. Often, those who experience a panic attack may develop a fear of dying, of loss of control, or of becoming insane.

While being anxious may be tolerable for many Chicanas, a panic attack is extremely frightening, as it is experienced physically, more than psychologically, at least initially.

■ Vignette #6: A case of panic attack

Julia, a twenty-six–year-old, second-generation Chicana, worked as a driver for an agricultural company in Central California. She began to experience symptoms of anxiety—nervios—when her husband, Miguel, began adjustment proceedings to legalize his undocumented status. A few weeks prior to her first panic attack, Julia and Miguel had been to see their attorney, who explained that Miguel would need to leave the United States and seek a pardon and waiver in Ciudad Juárez.

Given the current immigration laws (Hing 2004; Cervantes, Mejia, and Guerrero Mena 2010), Miguel might have to remain in Mexico for at least a few weeks, and if the pardon was denied, he could be punished and barred from reapplying for a visa to enter the United States for as long as ten years. Julia and Miguel agreed that they would take the chance and apply for a pardon and waiver of inadmissibility, since Miguel was no longer eligible to drive or work, and the couple needed his income to support their two small children and themselves.

While driving for work one day, Julia began to experience shortness of breath and chest pains. Her vision became blurred and she pulled over, as she believed she was having a heart attack. She began to shake uncontrollably and managed to contact her employer, who sent out an ambulance. In the emergency room Julia was diagnosed as having had a panic attack. Julia was ashamed that she was going crazy and that she was not the strong woman she needed to be to handle the challenges that lay ahead. Both Julia and Miguel were relieved to learn that her symptoms were caused by a panic attack, which was not unusual in cases of such severe stress. She was not "crazy" and could derive benefit from medication, particularly as she was afraid to drive but needed to because she was the only one working at the time. She understood that her "nervios" became too much in the face of such problems and affected her body. Prayer, teas, and an anxiolytic would help her regain balance.

Posttraumatic Stress Disorder

Posttraumatic stress disorder, first identified in combat veterans and survivors of natural disasters, is a syndrome involving the sequelae of directly experiencing or witnessing severe trauma (whether or not physical injury has occurred). The diagnosis can be used when a person has experienced, has witnessed, or has been confronted with an unusually traumatic event that involved actual or threatened death or serious physical injury to the person or to others, *and* as a result the individual felt intense horror, fear, or helplessness. Rape, childhood physical and sexual abuse, witnessing family violence, experiencing intimate partner violence, all can result in the development of PTSD (Diaz and Lieberman 2010; Rodriguez et al. 2008; van der Kolk 1997, 2005).

Trauma affects the mind, body, and spirit of an individual. Thus, symptoms may be cognitive (difficulty with memory, concentration, and the ability to anticipate danger, which can result in a higher risk for subsequent victimization), emotional (as in depressed mood or anxiety disorders), or physical (aches and pains with no apparent physical cause, difficulty breathing), and relational. Sexually abused women typically experience difficulty with sexuality in intimate relationships and may avoid dating as a result of fear of intimacy with potential partners (Flores-Ortiz 2004; Herman 1992).

In the case of sexual victimization, women invariably feel dirty, guilty, and ashamed. Often, perpetrators of sexual violence tell the women that they "asked for it" by calling attention to themselves, being alone, dressing "provocatively," or being exotic. Women of color often are the targets of sexual violence as a result of displaced rage by males of color, and because they are socially devalued and subject to stereotyping by media and popular culture as either passive and virginal or exotic and licentious (Hardy and Laszloffy 2005). Thus, when they are victimized, women are susceptible to accepting blame and feeling shame (Flores 2003).

When the abuse occurs in the family, adult perpetrators often tell the victimized children that they are special and loved more than those who are not abused. In some instances, children are threatened with harm to siblings or parents if they disclose the abuse, and are thereby silenced (Flores-Ortiz 1997a). Cloé Madanes (1990; Madanes, Keim, and Smelser 1997), a family therapist who specializes in the treatment of abuse in the family, argues that when a child is violated within the home, a distorted connection is formed between love, sex, and violence that often results in PTSD *and* increased risk to succumb to abusive relationships in adulthood. Likewise, childhood victimization and adult trauma increase the risk of substance abuse among women (Champion et al. 2001; Flores-Ortiz 1997b, 1998, 2003; Lipsky et al. 2004). The shame, pain, and hopelessness resulting from abuse may create a belief in the victimized woman that she is not worthy of being treated fairly, particularly if her perpetrator is an intimate partner who blames her for his violent actions and his lack of control (Johnson 2008; Johnson and Leone 2005).

A victimized woman's self-esteem is eroded by violence, lack of support, and being held responsible for her own victimization. This damage is often exacerbated when she discloses the abuse and is not believed or when she presses charges and is revictimized by the justice system (Almeida and Lockard 2005; Flores 2003; Lipsky et al. 2006).

Traumatized individuals repeatedly relive the event in at least one of these ways: intrusive, distressing recollections (thoughts, images); repeated

distressing dreams; flashbacks, hallucinations, or illusions; feeling or acting as if the event were recurring; marked mental distress in reaction to
internal or external cues that symbolize or resemble some part of the event
or physiological reactions in response to these cues, which may be similar
to panic attack, such as rapid heartbeat, sweaty palms, and elevated blood
pressure.

As a result of the distress generated by the symptoms, the affected individual repeatedly avoids situations that are related to or remind her of
the trauma. She may experience numbing of general responsiveness—she
freezes up and feels paralyzed to act (absent before the traumatic event).
As a result, she tries to avoid feelings, thoughts, or conversations concerned
with the traumatizing event and tries to avoid activities, people, or places
that recall the trauma. She may show a marked loss of interest or participa-
tion in activities that were previously important or enjoyable. In addition,
the traumatized person feels detached or isolated from people; she experiences restriction in ability to love or feel strong emotions and at times feels
that her life will be brief or unfulfilled (that is, she is not fit for marriage,
having children, or obtaining a good job, for example). The individual
affected by PTSD often has symptoms of hyperarousal that were not present before the traumatic event: insomnia (initial or interval), poor concentration, angry outbursts or irritability, and excessive vigilance (American
Psychiatric Association 2000; Herman 1992).

Ironically, the symptoms do not usually develop immediately after the
traumatic event; thus, the symptoms may become even more frightening
as a connection may not be made between the event and the distress experienced later. In some instances the traumatized individual may experience
feelings of guilt or personal responsibility (I should have prevented what
happened) or have survivor's guilt, particularly in situations where others
died or were seriously hurt.

The relationship between gender and sexual violence and the development of PTSD has been well established (Almeida 1998; Almeida et al. 1994;
Herman 1992; van der Kolk 1994, 1997, 2005). Witnessing or experiencing
family violence often results in PTSD and depression among women. In
my earlier work I documented the emotional, psychological, physical, and
spiritual impact of rape, incest, and IPV on Chicanas and Latinas (Bauer
et al. 2000; Flores 2003; Flores-Ortiz 1993a, 1997b, 1998, 1999, 2004, 2005a
and b; Flores-Ortiz, Esteban, and Carrillo 1994; Rodriguez et al. 1998). In
our work with Mexican women and Chicanas, Enriqueta Valdez Curiel

and I (Flores and Valdez Curiel 2009) collected their narratives of family violence. Chicanas expressed the desperation, grief, and soul wounding that result from experiencing betrayal by family members. Julia, a twenty-five-year-old Chicana, asked, "If you cannot trust your father, your brothers, to respect and honor you, who can you trust?"

The indigenous explanatory model holds that spiritual disorders are rooted in violations of the tonal—the spirit. When all aspects of the person are in harmony with the inner self and the universe, the soul is intact. The spiritual self, the aura that surrounds us, is most vulnerable to trauma. By our diet, habits, and attitudes, we can create an aura that is strong or one that is weak and full of holes. Experiencing a frightening or traumatic event can lead to soul loss, a state in which we do not feel fully present or as if we are not really ourselves; we may feel something is missing because the soul has been violated (Avila and Parker 2000). In the western explanatory model, soul loss can be described as dissociation. The soul wounding that results from abuse in childhood or adulthood, IPV, rape, and other forms of trauma can result in the fright of susto or *espanto*.

According to mestizo psychology, one can heal quickly from susto if the body, mind, and spirit are strong. Espanto is a more serious form of susto that is caused by seeing a ghost, by being awakened suddenly from deep sleep before the spirit has returned to the body, or through experiencing major trauma. Treatment entails limpias, rituals, and soul retrieval (Avila and Parker 2000).

While biomedical explanations for the onset of PTSD refer to excessive levels of cortisol being released as a result of the traumatic event, and the cultural explanatory model may attribute the distress to soul loss, the physiological, cognitive, and emotional symptoms of PTSD, susto, and espanto are similar. Healing from these experiences requires time and multiple treatments that can include medication, bodywork, and psychotherapy if treated from a western perspective, and cleansings, prayers, and other rituals if treated from a cultural perspective. Both forms of treatment in combination may be most effective for individuals who hold a mixed explanatory model, as is often the case with Latinos (Haan et al. 2003).

Among Chicanas with a history of violence, whether in childhood, adolescence, or adulthood, mood and anxiety disorders are more prevalent. For women in intimately violent relationships, the cultural mandate to remain in the marriage and try harder to make things work, economic dependency, and fear are the major deterrents to leaving the relationship

(Flores and Valdez Curiel 2009; Rodriguez et al. 2009). However, PTSD and major depression also paralyze, thus limiting the woman's ability to seek help or to disclose the abuse. Given the high prevalence of IPV among Chicanas (see Lown and Vega 2001), it is imperative to assess for mood disorders among women who are in abusive relationships as well as evaluate for IPV in women who present with mood or anxiety disorders.

■ Culture-Bound Syndromes

The growth of the Latino population in the United States led to the inclusion of "culture-bound syndromes" in the *DSM-IV-TR*. Among these, ataque de nervios (ADN) is the most prevalent, particularly among Puerto Rican and other Caribbean women (Lewis-Fernandez et al. 2002; Keough et al. 2009; Salgado de Snyder, Diaz-Perez, and Ojeda 2000), but also present among Chicanas. Ataque de nervios is an acute, fit-like exacerbation of nervios; it may include uncontrollable shouting, attacks of crying, trembling, heat in the chest rising to the head, and verbal or physical aggression. It is often present among women who also experience major depression, dysthymia, agoraphobia, phobic disorder, and panic disorder (Guarnaccia et al. 2010).

Somatization is another culture-bound syndrome (with greater incidence among Puerto Ricans and Mexicans than other Latinos), since Latinos are less likely to separate between mind and body than are Anglos (Avila and Parker 2000); therefore, they are likely to experience emotional distress physically. Somatization is a psychiatric condition marked by multiple physical or somatic symptoms serious enough to interfere significantly with a person's ability to perform important activities, such as work, school, or family and social responsibilities, or to lead the person experiencing the symptoms to seek medical treatment. However, no medical cause is found to explain the symptoms. Somatization may be less stigmatizing than suffering from an emotional or psychiatric disorder, which may contribute to its higher incidence among individuals from cultures where emotional or psychiatric problems are highly stigmatized (Escobar et al. 1987; Flores, Zelman, and Flores 2012).

The physical manifestation may represent an idiom of distress or be symbolic of the spiritual or emotional pain being experienced. Backaches from "carrying the weight" or financial burden of a family, headaches from "thinking too much," body aches and pains associated with depression may be reported to a primary care physician because they are not recognized as having a psychological or emotional origin.

■ Psychotic Disorders

Psychotic disorders are serious psychiatric illnesses that alter a person's ability to think clearly, make good judgments, respond emotionally, communicate effectively, understand reality, and behave appropriately. In severe cases, the affected person may have difficulty staying in touch with reality and may be unable to meet the ordinary demands of daily life. While the specific causes of psychotic disorders are unknown, research points to a hereditary and genetic predisposition, which can develop into a disorder if environmental factors are present or occur, such as stress, major life changes, or drug use. In the case of schizophrenia, however, an imbalance of dopamine, a neurotransmitter, is implicated in the development of hallucinations and delusions (National Institute of Mental Health 2005).

Psychotic disorders usually are treatable with medication, if diagnosed accurately. There are different types of psychotic disorders; the most common and better known is schizophrenia, which causes changes in behavior and delusions (false beliefs) and hallucinations that last longer than six months and impair the ability to attend school or work and adversely affect social functioning. Schizophrenia has a worldwide prevalence of about 1 percent.

Chicanos are likely to describe the symptoms of schizophrenia as locura. This is a highly stigmatized disorder, as it is often not well understood by families (Breitborde, Lopez, and Kopelowicz 2010; Lopez and Guarnaccia 2000). Onset is typically in late adolescence and young adulthood, and family members may confuse the problematic behavior with malacrianza, that is, rebelliousness or disrespect. A number of community education campaigns have been developed both in the United States and in Mexico to increase the awareness and understanding of psychotic disorders and thereby increase the likelihood of earlier detection and treatment (see Lopez et al. 2009). Once a person is diagnosed, Latino families generally rally in support of that individual and seek treatment.

Other psychotic disorders include schizoaffective disorder, which includes symptoms of both schizophrenia and a mood disorder, such as depression or bipolar disorder. Schizophreniform disorder is another psychotic disorder with symptoms similar to schizophrenia, but lasting only between one and six months. A brief psychotic disorder may occur in response to a very stressful life event, for example, the death of a family member, and be characterized by a short period of psychotic behavior. The symptoms typically abate within one month. A delusional disorder is also brief, with symptoms persisting at least one month. It may be difficult for the family to recognize the disorder, as the affected individual may have delusions of real-life situations that are plausible, for example, being followed, having a disease, or being the object of envy, jealousy, or political persecution. A shared psychotic disorder, commonly referred to as "folie à deux," occurs when a person develops false beliefs or delusions in the context of a relationship with another person equally affected. This can occur among family members or hospital patients. Substance-induced psychotic disorder is a condition caused by the use of or withdrawal from drugs such as alcohol, methamphetamine, or crack cocaine. Abuse or withdrawal from these drugs may cause hallucinations, delusions, or confused speech (flight of ideas). Paraphrenia is a type of schizophrenia that starts late in life and occurs in the elderly population.

It is important to recognize psychotic disorders early, as some may in fact be caused by medical conditions, such as a head injury or a brain tumor, that can be fatal if undetected or improperly treated.

■ Substance Abuse Disorders

Epidemiological studies find that Latinas in general and Mexican-origin women in particular are mostly alcohol abstainers and evidence lower incidence of drug abuse when compared to Chicano or Mexican men, or to European American women. However, with increased acculturation, Chicanas and Latinas consume more alcohol and are at greater risk for substance abuse disorders (Alegria et al. 2007; Caetano et al. 2010).

According to the Substance Abuse and Mental Health Services Administration (US Dept. of Health and Human Services 2009), the primary substances abused by Chicanas seeking treatment were methamphetamine (34 percent), alcohol (22.6 percent), marijuana/hashish (15.6 percent), cocaine/crack (12 percent), and heroin (11.6 percent).

The identified risk factors for Chicanas include acculturative stress, history of trauma (in particular childhood abuse and adult intimate partner violence) (Lipsky and Caetano 2007), identity confusion, and sexual identity problems (including the stigma of being bisexual, lesbian, or transgendered).

In addition, Latina substance abusers tend to be younger, have fewer years of education, and be unemployed (Caetano et al. 2010). In California, over 16 percent of Latinas seeking admission for alcohol or drug treatment were younger than nineteen years of age; 36.9 percent were between the ages of nineteen and twenty-nine years of age, and 25.1 percent were between thirty and thirty-nine. About 45 percent of Latinas remain in treatment for less than one month (Caetano et al. 2010).

The *DSM-IV-TR* distinguishes between substance abuse and substance dependence. Substance dependence, commonly known as addiction or chemical dependency, is defined as the core behavior of those who misuse substances. Dependence includes behavioral, physiological, and cognitive symptoms. In the case of substance dependence the user has taken a substance frequently enough to produce psychological or emotional distress or impaired functioning (at school, work, or in family relationships), as well as certain behavioral characteristics ranging from denial and hiding of the use to criminal behavior. Dependence is found in connection with all classes of drugs (except caffeine) and does not necessarily have a recreational origin; it can develop from medicinal use (for example, painkillers).

■ Vignette #7: "I loved alcohol more than my own *hija* (daughter)"

Sofia, a fifty-eight-year-old, second-generation Chicana, sought therapy to repair her relationship with her daughter. Sofia had been diagnosed with cancer the previous year. As she put it, "The cancer sentence got me to stop drinking after forty years of alcohol abuse." Sofia associated her alcohol abuse with internal conflicts regarding her sexuality. Sofia always knew she was lesbian; however, being the daughter of traditional immigrant parents, she tried to live a "straight life." She married and had a daughter, Jenny. However, she was unhappy living a double life and pretending to be someone she was not; thus, she coped by drinking. She developed alcohol dependence and realized that she could not be a good enough mother; she left her husband and daughter. Jenny was six years old. Sofia had visitation rights; however, her daughter complained that most of the time she visited her mom, her mother was drunk. Jenny recounted the terror she experienced while her mother drove drunk and exposed her to multiple girlfriends and drunken rages. Jenny was full of resentment because her mother had chosen alcohol over her.

Sofia knew that her drinking had led to a life of hurt for her daughter. She acknowledged that she could not quit drinking. She never missed a day of work, however, and was always able to provide for herself. Ana resented this as well. How could her mother stay sober for work, but not for her? When diagnosed with cancer and given a poor prognosis, Sofia sought help to repair her relationship with her daughter before she died. She did not want her daughter to have guilt. She wanted to be accountable and give her daughter an opportunity to express her pain.

Neither woman fully understood the nature of alcohol dependence. Jenny needed to understand the social and historical context in which her mother grew up. Sofia had received minimal support for her biculturality or her sexuality during adolescence. She had grown up with a father "who drank," and she learned early to cope through alcohol use. Perhaps as a combination of genetic predisposition, exposure to her father's drinking, and a peer system that abused alcohol, Sofia became alcohol dependent. She saw herself as a woman of little worth—despite her talent and education— because she was marginalized since childhood for her indigenous looks, her mild accent, and her sexuality. She gave up her daughter, as she did not believe she could be a good enough mother. She had accepted her family's belief that "lesbians could not be good parents."

In turn Jenny did not understand why her mother left her. She longed for her mother's love and presence. The years of her mother's substance dependence led to resentment and "a cold heart" toward her mother. She herself became a single parent and turned all her love to her son. She struggled with depression and anxiety for most of her young adulthood.

During their therapy sessions, where the women engaged in *pláticas*, they discovered that despite their estrangement, they had remained connected by pain. While Jenny remained ambivalent about her mother's desire for reconnection, she began to understand the nature of alcohol dependence and to accept her mother's love. Jenny began to understand the gift her mother offered—to develop a healthy adult relationship before her mother became absent through death.

A characteristic of dependence is that the use of substances is maladaptive; its use (perhaps to cope with other problems) only makes things worse for the user, as well as the user's relatives and friends. There is a repetitive pattern to the use that becomes a habit. To be considered dependent on a substance, the use has caused distress or impairment in a single twelve-month period. The substance use must be serious enough to interfere with the user's life (missed work, school, arrest for driving under the influence) or loss of parental custody, as was the case with Sofia, who gave up her daughter because she could not stop drinking.

■ Vignette #8: "I will never be weak"

As stated, childhood histories of trauma are a risk factor for adult substance dependence. Jennifer, a twenty-nine-year-old Chicana, witnessed extreme family violence. Her father routinely beat her mother; on one occasion the beating was so severe that her mother was left in a coma. Her father was then incarcerated for seven years. As an adult, Jennifer was remanded to anger management for her aggressive behavior toward co-workers. She described herself as a *pelionera* (a fighter) in high school. She identified with her aggressive father, not with her "weak" mother, and utilized alcohol to "feel happy." While she denied that her drinking was a problem, she often had to rely on her mother to take care of her one-year-old son because "she had trouble waking up" after a night of drinking.

Jennifer had to come to terms with her "drinking problem" when her mother threatened to report her to Child Protective Services and have her son removed from her custody. Jennifer was adamant that she could experience happiness only when she drank. The rest of the time she "went to a very dark place." Through "talking therapy" Jennifer came to see the connection between her drinking and the pain accumulated from years of bearing witness to her father's violence and her mother's pain. She decided to attempt sobriety in order to be more present with her son and respond to his emotional needs as well as take care of her own in more constructive ways. She decided to break the chain of violence, absence through alcohol, and self-abuse that pervaded her family history.

Substance abuse is a residual category for patients whose substance use produces problems but does not meet criteria for dependence.

Substance intoxication is an acute clinical condition resulting from recent overuse of a substance. The diagnosis can apply to individuals who use a drug only once. Substance intoxication symptoms tend to be substance-specific; however, there are certain common themes, among them motor incoordination or agitation, loss of ability to sustain attention, impaired memory, reduced alertness (drowsiness, stupor, or even coma), and specific effects on the autonomic nervous system (dry mouth, heart palpitations, gastrointestinal symptoms, changes in blood pressure), as well as mood changes (depression, euphoria, anxiety, and others). Substance intoxication can be a common occurrence among teenagers and college-aged women who begin to experiment with alcohol.

Substance withdrawal is a collection of symptoms, specific for the class of substance, that develop when a person who has frequently used a substance discontinues or markedly reduces the amount used. All substances produce withdrawal symptoms, which can result in emotional distress or impairment in work, social, or other functioning. The symptoms of withdrawal include alteration in mood (anxiety, irritability, or depression), abnormal motor activity (restlessness, immobility), sleep disturbance (insomnia or hypersomnia), and other physical problems (fatigue, changes in appetite).

Historically, Chicanos have perceived substance dependence as reflecting a weakness of character, and not as a disease. Latino cultures have been described as tolerant of male alcohol abuse but not of drug use or abuse (see chapter 4) (Lipsky and Caetano 2007). Attitudes are particularly negative toward women who abuse alcohol and other drugs, as they are perceived as sexually loose and, if they are parents, as bad mothers (as in Sofia's and Jennifer's cases) (Mora 2003).

Some scholars have equated opiate use and alcohol abuse with slow suicide (Bernal and Flores-Ortiz 1990). Other scholars have noted how alcohol was used as a tool of colonization in Mesoamerica, resulting perhaps in a great predisposition to dependence among mestizos (Cervantes and Felix-Ortiz 2004). Furthermore, whether substance-dependent Chicanas began to use alcohol or other drugs to cope with childhood victimization, or adolescent identity conflicts, or adult losses or traumatic experiences, once dependency developed, the women became *unable* to stop the substance use on their own. Moreover, the losses associated with long-term substance dependence—those of health, custody of children, work, status, family support—in turn can serve as risk factors that deter sobriety and propitiate relapse. Sofia, for example, often drank because she missed her daughter. However, when her daughter came to visit, she could not wait for Jenny to leave so that she could drink again.

Given the similarity of symptomatology between substance dependence and the mood disorders *and* the fact that they often co-occur, it is critical to assess for use of substances in clients who present with a mood disorder, and for mood disorder in substance-dependent individuals. Likewise, the sociocultural factors that contribute to substance abuse and dependence must be understood in order to develop culturally attuned treatments.

In the case of women with substance dependence problems, the risks of incarceration due to illegal activities (buying or selling drugs, exchanging sex for drugs, theft or robbery) and losing custody of their children are very high. In fact, most Chicanas in prison are incarcerated for drug offenses or for being the partners of men who abuse or sell drugs (Institute on Women and Criminal Justice 2009). Likewise, women with substance dependence are at greater risk for experiencing physical and sexual violence (Cervantes and Felix-Ortiz 2004), as they often are unable to protect themselves or are more likely to be involved with substance-abusing social networks.

The negative consequences of substance abuse and dependence are great for women, in particular the loss of child custody; thus, many women do not seek treatment voluntarily, to prevent losing their children. While the creation of gender-specific services for women has increased access to treatment, policies that punish women for abusing alcohol and drugs continue to create barriers to services. Moreover, recognition of the sociocultural factors that contribute to women's substance abuse and dependence has resulted in increased awareness of the need for gender- and culturally specific treatment models that are trauma informed; that is, treatment efforts should consider the role of gender and experiences of trauma in the onset and course of the addiction (Covington 2008).

◼ Summary

The threats to the emotional well-being of Chicanas are largely structural; moreover, social and cultural factors also must be taken into consideration. Discrimination, marginalization, microaggressions and othering, pressures to acculturate to an often rejecting culture, and lack of understanding from immigrant parents and relational challenges rooted in acculturative stressors constitute risk factors for mood and anxiety disorders.

The multiple forms of injustice that women experience from both strangers and loved ones, especially violence and substance abuse *within* the home, threaten their lives and psychological health. Chicanas generally become substance dependent as the result of exposure to or experience of violence, microaggressions, and multiple forms of injustice. They may begin to use alcohol and other drugs in adolescence, and if they continue, by middle adulthood this use will have resulted in dependence and family, social, and emotional problems. Whether understood or experienced as spiritual, relational, emotional, or behavioral, a Chicana's recovery from the pain caused by injustice requires healing of her soul, mind, heart, and body.

■ Discussion Questions

1. What are some cultural factors that influence the development of depression among Chicanas?

2. What is the emic equivalent of PTSD?

3. What educational strategies may prevent substance dependence among Chicanas?

4. What are some of the similarities between PTSD and susto?

5. What are some cultural protective factors that may deter mood disorders among Chicanas?

■ Note

1. The eleven mood disorders include: bipolar 1 and 2, bipolar disorder not otherwise specified (NOS), cyclothymic disorder, depressive disorder not otherwise specified (NOS), depression, dysthymic disorder, major depressive disorder, mood disorder due to a general medical condition (such as diabetes), mood disorder not otherwise specified, and substance-induced mood disorder.

■ Suggested Readings

Almeida, Rhea. "Has the Focus on Multiculturalism Resulted in Inadequate Attention to Factors Such as Gender, Social Class, and Sexual Orientation?" In *Controversial Issues in Multiculturalism,* ed. Diane De Anda, 261–75. Boston: Allyn and Bacon, 1997.

———. *Transformations of Gender and Race: Family and Developmental Perspectives.* New York: Haworth, 1998.

Almeida, Rhea, and Judith Lockard. "The Cultural Context Model: A New Paradigm for Accountability, Empowerment, and the Development of Critical Consciousness against Domestic Violence." In *Domestic Violence at the Margins: Readings on Race, Class, Gender, and Culture,* ed. N. Sokoloff, 301–20. New Brunswick, NJ: Rutgers University Press, 2005.

Almeida, Rhea, Theresa Messineo, Rosemary Woods, and Robert Font. "Violence in the Lives of the Racially and Sexually Different: A Public and Private Dilemma."

In *Expansions of Feminist Family Therapy through Diversity,* ed. Rhea Almeida, 99–134. London: Psychology Press, 1994.

Champion, Jane Dimmitt, Rochelle N. Shain, Jeanna Piper, and Sondra T. Perdue. "Sexual Abuse and Sexual Risk Behaviors of Minority Women with Sexually Transmitted Diseases," *West Journal of Nursing Research* 23, no. 3 (April 2001): 241–54.

Denner, Jill, and Bianca L. Guzmán, eds. *Latina Girls: Voices of Adolescent Strength in the United States.* New York: New York University Press, 2006.

Espin, Oliva. *Latina Realities: Essays on Healing, Migration and Sexuality.* Boulder, CO: Westview Press, 1997.

Flores, Yvette G. *"La Salud*: Latina Adolescents Constructing Identities, Negotiating Health Decisions." In *Latina Girls,* ed. Jill Denner and Bianca Guzmán, 199–211. New York: New York University Press, 2006.

———. "Parenting." In *Encyclopedia Latina: History, Culture, and Society in the United States*, ed. Ilan Stavans, 316–22. Danbury, CT: Scholastic Library, 2005a.

———. "Rape." In *Latinas in the United States: An Historical Perspective*, ed. Virginia Sanchez Korrol, Vicki L. Ruiz, and Carlos Cruz, 611–13. Bloomington: Indiana University Press, 2005b.

Flores-Ortiz, Yvette. "Psychotherapy with Chicanas at Midlife: Cultural/Clinical Considerations." In *Racism in the Lives of Women*, ed. Jeanne Adelman and Gloria Enguídanos, 251–60. New York: Haworth Press, 1995.

———. "Re/membering the Body: Latina Testimonies of Social and Family Violence." In *Violence and the Body: Race, Gender, and the State*, ed. Arturo J. Aldama, 347–59. Bloomington: Indiana University Press, 2003.

Gallegos-Castillo, Angela. "La Casa: Negotiating Family Cultural Practices, Constructing Identities." In *Latina Girls,* ed. Jill Denner and Bianca Guzmán, 44–58. New York: New York University Press, 2006.

4

Los Hombres

The Negotiation of Grief and Pain

As early as childhood, Chicanos may experience microaggressions and "daily indignities" (Franklin and Boyd-Franklin 2000; Sue 2010) that can attack the body, mind, and heart. Chicano boys often are problematized in the community, school, and even in the home as disobedient, willful, conduct disordered, and aggressive (Aguirre-Molina and Betancourt 2010). As Hardy and Laszloffy (2005) have demonstrated, men of color encounter devaluation, loss of community, and dehumanization of loss, which for Chicanos have both historical and contemporary roots. In his classic book *El espejo enterrado* (The buried mirror), Carlos Fuentes (1998) describes the Mexican as he who was born at the precise moment of his death. Octavio Paz (1962) and Rogelio Diaz-Guerrero (1975) described the psychology of Mexican men as embodying both the colonizer and the colonized. Thus, depending on his identification and the degree of internalization of negative stereotypes, a Chicano can embody the victim and/or the perpetrator of aggression. Chicano men carry that legacy on their shoulders. They may also carry the scars of historical trauma. Furthermore, the complicated history of Mexicanos/Chicanos in the United States can further impact the sense of self and the mental health of Chicanos. Experiences of discrimination and marginalization as a result of minority status can produce psychiatric distress (Aguirre-Molina, Borrell, and Vega 2010; Finch, Kolody, and Vega 2000; Williams and Jackson 2005), particularly for those men who remain in the margins of society or become part of the urban underclass (Portes, Fernandez-Kelly, and Haller 2005; Rumbaut 1994).

This chapter explores the gender socialization of Mexicano/Chicano men of various social classes and the role of cultural values, "minority status," and histories of oppression on their experience and expression of emotional and spiritual distress. In addition, contemporary self-empowerment and healing efforts that emerged in the 1970s are discussed as potential avenues to strengthen the mental health of Chicanos.

■ Chicanos and Mental Health

As stated in earlier chapters, the growth of the Latino population has resulted in greater attention to health disparities and the prevalence of psychiatric disorders among Latino subgroups (Alegria et al. 2007, 2008; Vega et al. 2010). Available epidemiological data regarding the mental health of the three major Latino groups (Puerto Rican, Cuban, and Mexican American/Chicano) indicate different lifetime prevalence estimates. For example, the LA-ECA study (1983–84) found a 3 percent prevalence estimate for depression, 7.3 percent for phobia, 3 percent for alcohol, and 1 percent for panic disorder. In contrast, the MAPPS study (1994–96) found much higher rates for depression (9 percent) and lower ones for alcohol dependence (3.3 percent) among Mexican immigrants (Aguilar-Gaxiola et al. 2002). The rates were similar for phobia and panic. The National Latino and Asian American Study (NLAAS) (Alegria et al. 2004; Kessler and Merikangas 2005) found significantly higher rates of mental disorder among Chicanos than Mexican immigrants (Guarnaccia et al. 2010; Alegria et al. 2008). These authors concluded that the longer an immigrant resides in the United States, the more compromised his mental health may be. This was the case for both men and women.

Polo and Alegria (2010) compared the epidemiological data obtained through the NLAAS with that of non-Latino white men obtained with the National Comorbidity Survey Replication Study (NCS-R) (Kessler and Merikangas 2005). Latino and non-Latino white men were compared across various sociodemographic, structural, and "clinical characteristics, including lifetime and past-year rates of depressive, anxiety and substance use disorders" (183). Polo and Alegria found that Latino men in the NLAAS sample were younger than non-Hispanic white men in the NCRS sample; they also had lower educational attainment and lower household income, were twice as likely to be unemployed, and were three times as likely to lack health insurance as their non-Latino peers.

Polo and Alegria (2010) also noted that the lifetime prevalence rates of any disorder were not significantly different from those of non-Latino white men across the eleven psychiatric disorders they investigated. Among the Latino men, Mexican-origin men reported more acculturative stress.

In terms of psychiatric diagnosis, Alegria and her colleagues (2008) had established lifetime prevalence estimates for psychiatric distress to be 28.81 percent for Latinos and 30.2 percent for Latinas. For Mexican-origin males the estimates were 28.42 percent for lifetime, and 14.48 percent for past-year, psychiatric disorder. That is, over a fourth of Mexicans and Chicanos may experience a psychiatric disorder in their lifetime. Comparisons of prevalence rates across Chicanos of different generations found that third-generation men had higher prevalence estimates for lifetime psychiatric disorder than did first- or second-generation men, particularly with regard to depression, anxiety, and substance use. Moreover, second-generation men were more likely to have had depression and substance use disorders, as well as other psychiatric disorders, than were first-generation men, while third-generation men were more likely to have had lifetime substance use disorders.

English-dominant men appeared more at risk for psychiatric disorder than did bilingual or monolingual Spanish-speaking men, regardless of their level of education. Acculturative stress, poverty, microaggressions, and exposure to violence are the greatest predictors of psychiatric distress for men (Turner and Gil 2002). Moreover, third-generation men who may have greater acculturation to the dominant society and perhaps have experienced a weakening of family ties or adherence to traditional Mexican protective factors that are transmitted linguistically, may be even more at risk for substance use disorders (Gil and Vega 2010); or, as Portes and colleagues (2005) have found, segmented assimilation or downward assimilation may contribute to the higher rates of psychological distress among Chicano men when compared with European American men or Mexican immigrant men.

Overall, SAMHSA (US Department of Health and Human Services 2009) found only a 6.8 percent mental health treatment rate in the previous year for "Hispanics." As stated in the introduction, low service utilization is closely associated with structural barriers that limit access to services. Furthermore, gender plays a role in mental health service utilization, with men utilizing formal health care less frequently than women across ethnic and racial groups.

As with women, the way in which a Chicano understands and explains his emotional, physical, and spiritual distress will influence whether and from whom he seeks services. Alegria et al. (2007) found only a 25 percent utilization rate for psychologists and other non-physician mental health providers among US-born Latinos, and a 10 percent utilization rate for psychiatrists, compared to 19 percent and 15 percent respectively for the immigrant Latinos in their sample. That study also found greater use of physicians or medication by US-born than immigrant Latinos (38 percent vs. 32 percent). Interestingly, US-born Latinos reported greater use of prayer and spiritual practices than did immigrant Latinos (29 percent vs. 12 percent respectively).

Gender and Mental Health

The gender socialization of males is influenced by the family's generation, social class, and educational level. The formation of a male identity in adolescence also is nuanced by enculturation (the degree of cultural knowledge and identification provided by the parents) and acculturation (which is influenced in turn by the larger sociocultural context). As Quintana and Scull (2009) propose, the ethnic identity of Chicanos and other Latinos occurs within a context of marginalization. Thus, very early in their development males come to identify as men and as members of a marginalized social group.

A legacy of the Chicano Movement of the 1960s has been the struggle to form an ethnic identity that is whole and that embraces the indigenous, Spanish, and US cultural and historical legacies of Mexican-origin people while reformulating psychoanalytically based definitions of Mexicans as the traumatized, defeated children of the raped indigenous woman (Diaz-Guerrero 1975; Paz 1962). According to these authors, Mexican men and their Chicano brothers suffer from an inferiority complex due to the conquest and the genocide inflicted upon their indigenous ancestors. Thus, men can identify either with their "superior" European conqueror or their "inferior" indigenous ancestor. The psychic pain often is masked by hypermasculinity—the oft-misunderstood and maligned machismo, the quest for power and control over others in order to feel better—which can become abusive, by the numbing of the historical pain through alcohol abuse, or by adopting a stoic, inscrutable persona.

Jerry Tello (2008) offers an alternative formulation of Chicano identity. He reconstructs the pre-Columbian notions of masculinity as recorded in the Códice Florentino (Book VI) and Códices Matritences del Real Palacio (VI) and de la Real Academia (VIII) (47) and offers these as models for Chicano men. The codices describe the proper conduct for men, which was to be taught to young boys from childhood by their fathers and male elders. Tello notes that "at the base of the culture were direct teachings to reinforce a sense of respect and interconnectedness founded on spirituality" (46).

According to Tello (2008), to transform a boy into *un hombre noble* requires family members, especially parents and grandparents, to teach the child the values of the culture and the behaviors consonant with those values, including respect, loyalty, and the proper way to treat elders, women, and peers. Traditional cultures encourage the family to help build a solid moral foundation for the child, so that he will become a hardworking, stoic, and reliable man (Flores 2005a; Tello 2008).

What does it mean to be a man? Over the past twenty-three years of teaching Chicano and Latino students, I have collected the adjectives used by young men to describe the ideal Chicano. Some descriptors reflect traditional values: hardworking, respectful, strong, family oriented, loyal, faithful, collaborative, dominant, "a player," head of household. A few students included *heterosexual* as a descriptor of the ideal man. Other adjectives reflect a more contemporary value system: well balanced, partner, devoted, good father, activist, and *hombre de palabra* (a man of his word), along with the more traditional descriptors.

When asked from whom they learned these ideas about masculinity, students invariably reported hearing such expectations at home. Their mothers often told them how a man should be. They saw the example mirrored in their fathers, grandfathers, uncles, or older brothers. When asked if these attributes defined them, most young Chicano students in my classes indicated that these were ideals to which they aspired but often found difficult to attain, given the constant belittlement of Chicanos they saw, heard, and experienced in the media and the larger society. As college students, they saw themselves often as "the exception" that had made it to college or as the survivors of the multiple barriers and structural limitations faced by their immigrant families. The young men stated that they experienced acculturative stress from the time they entered elementary school and continued to face microaggressions on a daily basis at the university. Chicanos who were second- or third-generation still held traditional values, although some felt less connected to the culture that informed those values.

▪ Protective and Risk Factors

High school Chicanos interviewed for a larger study of health practices (Flores 2006) described countless experiences of discrimination and racism both at school and in the community. By the time they were ten years of age, many had concluded that they were part of a marginalized social group (Hurtado and Gurin 2004) and as such had begun to reject the dominant culture. Many of the youth expected to have a hard life, to be noticed only when perceived as a threat, and to remain invisible when they did positive things. Not surprisingly, many had begun to disengage from school and to internalize the negative attributes projected onto them. Few had discussed these experiences with family members or peers. However, they had recognized the stoicism of their fathers, uncles, and older brothers as a possible stance against continual marginalization.

What made the difference for high school and college students who were succeeding academically? A supportive family, teacher, or mentor, they invariably responded. What threatened their success the most? Not fitting in, fear of failure, lack of support from family or friends who did not understand their desire for education or who could not provide economic support. Above all, they noted, the "daily dose" of microaggressions wounded their souls and eroded their confidence. Many experienced daily indignities—being racialized, profiled, stereotyped, and objectified.

My own son, at the age of eleven, came home one day and said, "Mom, it finally happened." "What happened?" I asked. He responded, "I was walking to the bus stop from school, and a white lady saw me walking in her direction. She clutched her purse close to her chest and crossed the street in a hurry." My light-skinned, eleven-year-old son, a privileged child of a university professor, had known that this day would come—that he would be viewed as a potential criminal on the basis of his "Mexican" appearance. Whether the woman had feared him for being a young brown male or for being a teen, or even if she had not feared him at all, he perceived her behavior as rejecting of who he was. Such injuries to the soul of a young boy, if frequent in occurrence, can compromise his mental health and produce the type of rage that can lead to violence in adolescence and adulthood.

■ What Ails the Hearts, Bodies, and Minds of Chicano Men

According to the US Department of Justice (2008), nationwide 2002–4, youth of color were overrepresented in the detained population at 3.1 times the rate of white youth. Custody rates for Latino youth were 1.8 times that of their white counterparts. Adult Chicano and Latino males are incarcerated at much higher rates than European American males (Arévalo,

Bécares, and Amaro 2010). The primary transgressions for which adult Chicano males are incarcerated include crimes against property, robbery, and homicide. Many of these acts are alcohol-related and other drug-related offenses. Furthermore, most adult offenders first became involved in the criminal justice system as juveniles—often for petty offenses for which non-Latino youth more likely would receive probation (Aguirre-Molina and Betancourt 2010; Chávez Garcia 2012; Hardy and Laszloffy 2005).

Fire and Firewater

Hardy and Laszloffy (2005), among others, have shed light on what leads men of color to engage in acts of violence. Carrillo and Zarza and others have addressed the psychological impact of childhood victimization on Chicano men and the resultant substance misuse, depression, and violence. For many Chicanos, "firewater" becomes the salve for spiritual and emotional pain—for the fires that rage within—(Carrillo and Zarza 2008; Tello 2008).

■ Vignette #9: Rage and Pain

Sergio, a twenty-eight-year-old, second-generation Chicano, explains it this way.

> I was born in Califas and lived with my parents and younger brother and sister in San Jose. One day, Dad packed us all in his car and said we were going for a drive. He drove all the way to Michoacán. He left us with his mother. He said he would be back soon. Mom later learned that he had another old lady in San Jo, so he just dumped us in Mexico to make his new woman happy. He just threw away his family for a piece of ass. Mom became very depressed. My little brother and sister started school and cried every day, because they did not know Spanish. I knew some, but not enough to fit in at school. I was thirteen. On my first day in school, the other *vatos* (guys) called me a *pocho* [US-born Mexican] and told me to go back home. How ironic—at school in San Jo the white kids called me beaner and told me to go home. So here I was, supposedly at home, only to discover I did not have a home. So I stopped going to school. I found work at a car shop, learned the trade. I also learned to drink with the older guys. I was about sixteen when my dad showed up again and, without an explanation, said we were coming home—back to the States—without even an explanation, much less an apology.

I have to admit, I became a knucklehead. I did not go to school. I was so far behind I would never catch up. I tried not to be home either; my parents fought all the time. My old man continued his womanizing ways, and Mom would yell and throw things. My old man would leave, and she would cry and threaten to leave him; but she never did. The only thing my dad ever gave me was a little pocketknife, which I always had with me. One time I was riding in a car with a homeboy, and the police stopped us. With guns drawn, the cops came to the car and told us to get on the ground. I guess I was not fast enough, because the cop threw me to the ground and searched me. He found the pocketknife and arrested me for having a concealed weapon. I spent six months in juvie [juvenile hall]. Mom did not have money for a lawyer, and my dad went on about what a mess-up I was and how disappointed he was, etc.

I went to juvie as a scared sixteen-year-old and came out a thug. I was angry; all I could feel was rage. So I started drinking and beating up people; then I went into heroin and crack and meth and anything I could get my hands on. After my first incarceration I met my girl. She is mixed—Asian and Latina—she understands what it is like not to fit in. We've been through a lot together. Her parents hate me, but her dad gave me a job. We have a son who is seven and is my life. But I could not stay clean, man. I just could not stay clean. So I ended up locked up again. When I drink I cannot think or see. All I feel is the rage. So I got into a fight and nearly killed a guy. Three years in the pen. My girl left me; she found out she was pregnant when I got sentenced. So when I came out and wanted to see my kids, meet my daughter, she took me back. I am trying, man; I am trying. I work again for my girl's dad, and I am going to junior college, but I still mess up. I cheat on her. I need the thrill of a new woman, of meaningless sex that is good. If I cannot have the drugs, I need the sex. But I feel bad. I'm hurting my girl; I am not being a good dad; I am letting them down. I am letting myself down.

Sergio experienced the four aggravating factors that contribute to youth violence—devaluation, disruption or erosion of community, dehumanization of loss, and rage (Hardy and Laszloffy 2005). His father took his family to Mexico without explanation because he had started another relationship. Sergio was devalued at school in both Mexico and the United States. His communities and his sense of belonging were eroded. His losses were unrecognized and unmourned. He experienced injustice in the community, within the legal system, and at home. He learned to drink and coped through drug use and used violence to numb the pain. "I have become my worst enemy," he said. He keeps "messing up," not living up to his ideals of masculinity—of being a good partner and father. Instead, he repeats his father's pattern, in a self-destructive way. He abandons his family through incarceration and unhealthy relationships with women he does not love. He has internalized the victim and victimizer and oscillates between the two. He wants to heal his body, heart, and mind. He will need a lot of support—bridges and mentors to get and stay sober and to deal with the wreckage caused by his substance abuse (see Carrillo and Zarza 2008; Tello 2008) and to come to terms with his history, as well as remain consistent in his efforts to be the *hombre noble* he wants to be.

Intimate Partner Violence

While Sergio was not physically violent toward his partner, he was violent toward others while under the influence of alcohol. Chicanos who abuse their intimate partners often do so while under the influence or use the alcohol abuse as an explanation for "loss of control" (Flores and Valdez Curiel 2009). While most Mexican-origin men are cast as *machista* (men who engage in negative masculine behaviors, including the oppression of women), batterers, and abusers of women by society and even their families, not all Mexican-origin men have internalized that particular stereotype or explode in rage in the face of injustice. Those who do, however, often engage in what has been described as relational violence—the aggression between partners when they lack more appropriate coping mechanisms to deal with frustration (Johnson 2008).

Other Chicanos may engage in a pattern of intimate terrorism (Johnson 2008; Johnson and Leone 2005), where physical and sexual aggression represent two forms of violence designed to control and break down the partner's spirit, mind, and heart. Such forms of violence tend to be more lethal and severely damage the mental health of the women as well as that of the children in the home (see Carrillo and Zarza 2008; Flores-Ortiz, Esteban, and Carrillo 1994; Perilla et al. in press; Perilla et al. 2012). Boys and teens exposed to intimate partner violence are traumatized and may develop mood and anxiety disorders. Such exposure also increases the risk for conduct disorder and violence (Gil and Vega 2010).

In some of my earlier work (Flores-Ortiz, Valdez Curiel, and Andrade 2002), my colleagues and I explored the relationship between being a recipient and a perpetrator of relational violence and feelings toward the partner and the relationship. We found that men who used physical, verbal, or emotional violence against their female intimate partners or who experienced verbal aggression from them emotionally disengaged from the women. They turned "cold" in order to dehumanize their partner or to avoid confrontations. Women, however, tended to want to remain connected to their spouses despite the abuse. Men tried to flee emotionally; the women pursued. This often resulted in further acts of aggression between them. Women in these abusive relationships experienced depression (Flores, Valdez Curiel, and Fierro 2011).

Whether being involved in abusive relationships leads to depression or other psychiatric distress in men has not been studied with Chicanos or Mexican men. However, clinical experience with men who batter indicates that very often at the root of IPV is a profound depression and *desesperanza* (hopelessness) (Carrillo and Zarza 2008). Likewise, exposure to family and social violence in childhood can impair the neurobiology of the brain, which in turn impacts the ability to self-regulate, control aggression, or regulate mood (Ziegler 2002), as well as compromises the development of emotional attachment of babies and small children (Diaz and Lieberman 2010). Men with attachment disorders may be more prone to engage in IPV when their emotional needs are not met or when they experience microaggressions (Flores-Ortiz 2004).

Moreover, Chicano men who engage in intimate terrorism often experienced childhood victimization and endured the multiple forms of soul wounding discussed previously (Carrillo and Zarza 2008; Hardy and Laszloffy 2005). The violence toward their partners and children and their overwhelming need to control may be the result of the impotence experienced in childhood (see Carrillo and Zarza 2008; Flores-Ortiz 2004; Tello 2008 for further elaboration of these ideas).

■ Vignette #10: "It is just a cultural legacy"

Intimate partner violence occurs in all social strata. Joseph and Nancy sought couples therapy to deal with his "anger issues and impulse control problems," since his aggression was threatening their marriage. Joseph is an attorney, and his wife a physician. While they both engaged in heated altercations and verbal abuse, Joseph had pushed, shoved, and pinned Nancy to the wall on multiple occasions. Joseph loved his wife and did not want to hurt her. However, he grew up in a violent home, where his working-class immigrant father abused alcohol and often hit his wife and children. Joseph swore he would not be like his father. However, he had limited coping skills and low frustration tolerance, which is often the case in individuals who experience trauma in childhood (van der Kolk 1997; Ziegler 2002).

Nancy had grown up in a similar situation and had vowed never to be a victim. She described herself as a warrior. Joseph faced microaggressions at work on a daily basis, as the only Chicano attorney in a large, lucrative legal practice. They wanted to treat each other better and not repeat the patterns of their childhood with their children. During one difficult therapy session, Joseph stormed out of the office. Nancy stated, "There goes five hundred years of culture." Her explanatory model viewed his aggression and explosive behavior as rooted in historical factors—the reaction of men to the conquest of Mexico and the loss of Mexican land to the United States. As a result, she viewed his behavior as unchangeable, thus incurable. The focus of therapy included a reanalysis of that narrative; while acknowledging the painful legacy of colonization and genocide to the souls and psyches of mestizos, it was important to seek internal resources for survival and more adaptive ways to deal with their soul wounding. Joseph acknowledged that he needed outlets other than aggression toward his wife for the pain and frustration of being marginalized despite his education.

■ Psychological Impact of Microaggressions

Anderson J. Franklin and Nancy Boyd-Franklin (2000) and Derald Sue (2010) have identified the pernicious impact of microaggressions on the mental health of men of color. Franklin (2004) describes the challenges for African American men to reach manhood and succeed within a society that either renders them invisible or criminalizes them. The signs of what Franklin labels the invisibility syndrome include frustration, increased awareness of perceived slights, chronic indignation (which may be perceived by others as the man having "a chip on his shoulder"), pervasive discontent and disgruntlement, anger and internalized rage, immobilization and difficulty getting things done (which may appear as depression), questioning of his worth, disillusionment and confusion, feeling trapped and conflicted about his racial identity, loss of hope, depression, and substance abuse (10–11). Derald Sue articulates the ways in which Latinos are also made invisible or criminalized. Microaggressions at times are subtle and minimized by those who perpetrate them. The victims at times do not feel entitled to complain. Henry, a second-generation Chicano judge, once confided that he felt guilty for complaining about slights he endured.

> I am a judge, for heaven's sakes. How many Chicano judges do you know? I don't have the right to complain. My dad worked in a factory; my grandfather in the fields. My *suegro* (father-in-law) died of asbestos contamination. I don't have the right to feel aggrieved. But I do feel the pain of never being considered good enough, despite my degrees, my diplomas, my experience, my car, my home, my *gabacha* (Anglo) wife. . . .

Despite his success and achievements, Henry walked through life continually being reminded of his class and ethnic origins. When he walked into the courtroom wearing his robes, he was respected. In the courthouse, unless he wore a suit, he often was mistaken for the "only other Mexican, the janitor," he said. Henry did not use aggression as a coping mechanism. However, he drank after work "sometimes a little too much" to suppress the pain and anger of the daily indignities he experienced. He was afraid his family would consider him weak, so he never told them about his own wounding. He felt guilty for complaining, since every man in his family, and his working-class-origin European American wife's family as well, had been a blue-collar worker, and in Henry's view these men had endured much greater offenses than he did. According to Franklin (1997), men like Henry may appear stoic and disconnected from their intimate relationships; their emotional energy is spent on suppressing the anger that burns inside. They are at great risk for hypertension and heart disease, as well as explosions of rage, if there is no outlet for the anger and pain that accumulate over a lifetime of discrimination (Williams and Jackson 2005).

Henry could understand and voice his pain and offer a political analysis of his situation to "another professional," yet he felt ashamed at the disclosure. Working-class men often feel disentitled to complain about work-related injustice and do not understand completely their children's activism or fear for their children's safety. Working-class men may be less likely to voice their distress.

◼ Pain and Its Meaning

Arthur Kleinman (1988) proposes that moral pain—and I would add spiritual pain—is often disregarded by the medical profession, as such suffering is intangible and therefore assumed to have psychological roots. Pain for which a structural or organic cause cannot be found typically is considered to be psychosomatic, that is, to have emotional or psychiatric roots; consequently, it may be treated as less valid or important by both the patient and the physician. In the traditional Mexican explanatory model, pain can be manifested in the body irrespective of its cause or "location." Physical pain may have symbolic meaning for the afflicted. It may be easier to complain about back pain than to speak about feeling marginalized or about being unseen.

■ Vignette #11: "If I cannot work, I will be useless"

Mr. Lopez, a sixty-three-year-old janitor, was referred to psychotherapy by his primary care physician because he could not find the cause of Mr. Lopez's chronic back pain. The physician assumed that Mr. Lopez was malingering—faking illness to avoid work. Mr. Lopez had worked since age five, when he sold papers on the streets of Texas. Then he followed the crops with his family. He graduated high school and was drafted. After Vietnam, he began to work in building maintenance. He was offended that his doctor would accuse him of pretending to be sick. He was furious, and very sad. He also feared that if he could not return to work, his family economy would be devastated.

Mr. Lopez had worked almost his entire life. One day at work he tried to lift a desk, and he experienced tremendous pain. His back began to spasm, and he fell to the floor. One of his coworkers called an ambulance. At the hospital, Mr. Lopez underwent a number of exams. The company for which he worked laid him off shortly thereafter. Mr. Lopez's children encouraged him to file a claim and try to get worker's compensation. However, Mr. Lopez was afraid that if he did, the company would retaliate and take away his medical benefits. Mr. Lopez stated, "I learned young to be quiet and do the job; to not antagonize the *patrón* (boss); to not complain." His more-acculturated children were of a different mind and obtained an attorney for their father. Mr. Lopez was embarrassed, fearing that "people would believe he was after easy money."

Mr. Lopez's pain was real and represented a culmination of many years of backbreaking labor. His pain gave voice to the innumerable injustices he had experienced in life. At sixty-three he appeared ten years older;

he considered himself an old man. After six months without employment or benefits—as the medical doctor declared him fit to return to work and uninjured, but his company would not rehire him—Mr. Lopez was admitted to the emergency room with an apparent heart attack. In fact, he had experienced a panic attack (see chapter 3). His family brought him to therapy again, hoping this time he would accept treatment. Mr. Lopez was referred to a Chicano/Latino men's group, where he could explore the historical roots of his pain and find comfort in the community of other men of color. Over the course of several months, Mr. Lopez's pain abated, and he returned to work at a different company.

Few studies have documented the health needs of Chicano war veterans (Villa, Harada, and Huynh-Hohnbaum 2010; Ybarra 2004). Chicanos and Latinos have a long history of military service in the United States. In fact, they are overrepresented in the military. Most Latino veterans, especially those who served in Vietnam, have worse health indicators and greater levels of PTSD than European American veterans and other men of color who served. The rates of unemployment and substance abuse among them are high (Villa, Harada, and Huynh-Hohnbaum 2010).

Mr. Lopez did not want to speak about the Vietnam War; he did not see a connection between his back pain and panic attack and the other unreported symptoms of PTSD (hyperalertness, insomnia, intrusive memories) and his war experiences. He was drafted right out of high school and spent many years in the jungle. He came back disillusioned and depressed and never talked about the war. He did not use the services at the VA hospital, as he felt that "the government never did anything for me, except kill my dreams."

In the Latino men's group, Mr. Lopez was surprised to learn that his physical and emotional symptoms were related to his war experience. With the support of the men in the group, some of whom had Vietnam veteran fathers, he began to talk about the war experience and begin the process of healing from war trauma.

■ Depression

In men depression may not manifest as it does in women. Instead, men are more likely to act out—through aggression and substance abuse (Carrillo and Zarza 2008; Velasquez and Burton 2009). Consequently, male depression may be un- or under-diagnosed. An angry young man can be frightening to family and society. However, rarely is it asked, What lies underneath the rage? Mr. Lopez, Sergio, and many men who present with problems of chronic pain, substance dependence, or violence often have an underlying depression that has not been recognized.

The leading causes of death for Latino males aged sixteen to twenty-five are suicide, homicide, and accidents (National Center for Health Statistics 2012). Invariably, alcohol or other drugs are involved. Depression often co-occurs with substance dependence and is often at the root of suicide and other forms of violence. As stated earlier, school disengagement, family dysfunction, and parental absence due to working two or more jobs can leave young men adrift. As Tello (2008) and Carrillo and Zarza (2008) have noted, to negotiate successfully the transition to adulthood, young Chicanos need guides and mentors. When filled with despair as a result of continued devaluation, Chicanos may resort to suicide or engage in behaviors that can get them killed or that result in incarceration—where further dehumanization most likely will occur. Young men may also look for community in gangs, which can lead to a life of violence and early death, unless community interventions and family support can provide viable alternatives (Barrera et al. 2004).

Given the cultural and societal expectation that men be the providers, unemployment and underemployment can contribute to episodes of major depression in men who are not involved with the criminal justice system. The focus on work among working-class men, and the absence of employer-provided or affordable health insurance, often results in men neglecting their physical and emotional health (Homan, Homan, and Carrasquillo 2010). According to the US Census Bureau (2008), 33 percent of Hispanics are uninsured. The figures are higher for men who do seasonal work, who work as laborers, or who cannot afford to have health insurance costs taken out of their paychecks. Work-related injuries are high, particularly since most job categories that Chicanos fill—in construction and the service industry—are risky (accidents involving tools, cooking, cleaning with solvents, etc.). Yet even among professional men, health care utilization is low. The cultural value of being stoic and strong may contribute to male avoidance of doctor visits. When men do consult a physician, it is most often for a work-related injury or when symptoms have become very severe.

Velasquez and Burton (2009) indicate that Chicanos "are less likely to seek psychotherapy on their own or because of internal motivations" (181).

Instead, they will seek therapy when they have been court ordered, or referred by a physician, or "dragged in" by a family member, or threatened with leaving by a spouse or romantic partner, or when looking for a quick resolution to a problem, so they can get back to work or continue with their lives without the "problem" they are having difficulty managing on their own or that is causing emotional distress.

Most working-class urban Chicano men start to work young, usually in their late teens. Chicanos raised in semi-urban or rural areas may begin to contribute to the family economy much earlier, even in childhood, as families may follow the crops (as did Mr. Lopez's family). After twenty or so years of work, men may begin to experience chronic pain due to untreated or poorly treated back, neck, leg, and hand injuries. Such injuries may result in disability, and not being able to work often leads to anxiety and depression, because the man's identity is threatened when he is no longer the provider. Chronic pain often results in depression as well (Flores, Zelman, and Flores 2012), as was the case with Mr. Lopez.

◾ Illness and Disability

Middle-aged Chicanos have high rates of diabetes, heart disease, cardiovascular disease, and hypertension (Aguirre-Molina et al. 2010; Echeverria and Diez-Roux 2010). All of these conditions are highly comorbid with depression. If the man holds a traditional explanatory model, he may focus on treating the physical ailments and not the emotional/psychological ones. He may perceive his depression or anxiety as a sign of weakness and failure as a man.

◾ Vignette #12: "Ya no sirvo para nada"

Don Sebastian, a fifty-six-year-old Chicano from Texas says: *"Pos ya no sirvo para nada. La diabetes no me deja trabajar."* He says that because he cannot work as a result of diabetes-related complications (early stages of renal failure and impaired vision due to diabetic retinopathy), he feels useless. "I am good for nothing," he states. He viewed his symptoms of major depression as part of the diabetes and therefore as untreatable. When don Sebastian's college-educated daughter came home for a visit, she took him to his primary care physician and demanded a referral to a psychologist. Don Sebastian initially refused to go. "I am sick, not loco," he stated. So I recommended to his daughter that the whole family go see a psychologist together in order to shift the focus away from him and onto diabetes management.

Don Sebastian agreed to go once "if it would help [his] wife and daughter." It was important for him to save face, not to appear weak in front of his family. So the focus of treatment was on finding ways in which he could support the family without earning an income. The eldest daughter asked him to watch the grandchildren while she worked. This was agreeable and helped him exercise, an important aspect of diabetes management. Exercise also helps reduce symptoms of depression. Don Sebastian was willing to take antidepressants, but not to engage in "talking therapy." He insisted that talking about not working and how he felt would not help. *Necesito hacer algo, no estar hablando pendejadas* (I need to do something, not to be talking about stupid things). However, he continued attending family meetings, because it helped his wife and children. Over time, once he felt comfortable with the family therapy, be began to talk about his sadness over his declining health, and his fear of becoming totally dependent on his family rather than supporting them as he believed he *should*.

◼ Immigration Policies and Transnational Families

Changes in immigration policies, especially the Illegal Immigration Reform and Illegal Immigrant Responsibility Act of 1996 (Cervantes, Mejia, and Guerrero Mena 2010; Hing 2004) adversely impacted mixed-status families, that is, families where one parent and/or one or more children are legal permanent residents (LRP) or US citizens and others are undocumented. Criteria for gaining legal status after undocumented entry have become increasingly stringent (de la Torre et al. 2010). In order for the undocumented spouse to regain entry into the United States, he or she must file a pardon and waiver of inadmissibility; in most cases, the undocumented person must leave the United States to be interviewed in Ciudad Juarez, Mexico. As a result, couples and/or parents and children become separated, sometimes for months and even years. Such separations are fraught with economic, emotional, and psychological distress (Cervantes, Mejia, and Guerrero Mena 2010).

Among various criteria that must be met for the unauthorized immigrant to be eligible for a waiver is that the LRP or citizen spouse would experience "extreme hardship"—hardship that is unusual or beyond that which would be expected—from the spouse's deportation or inadmissibility back into the United States (de la Torre et al. 2010; Hing 2004). Such hardship may be health related, including preexisting emotional or psychiatric problems. Consequently, psychologists increasingly are called upon to conduct psychological evaluations and render expert opinions (see Cervantes, Mejia, and Guerrero Mena 2010).

For Chicanos such separations are particularly painful when their spouses are undocumented, as they are put in a position of either keeping the children for the duration of the adjustment proceedings while the wife/mother is in Mexico or being separated from both the wife and children indefinitely. Moving to Mexico with the family generally is not an option for male spouses, as they have to remain in the United States to work to support two households. The emotional toll on these men often goes undocumented and untreated. The increasing drug-related violence and social insecurity in Mexico add to the distress created by separation, as the men fear for the safety of their families.

■ Vignette #13: "I risked my life for my country, and this is the thanks I get"

Julian is a thirty-eight-year-old, third-generation Chicano, a veteran of the first Gulf War. When he returned from the Gulf, he met and fell in love with Yesenia, a young Mexican woman. She had been brought to the United States as a toddler by her parents. She was unaware that she was undocumented, until she was fifteen years old and wanted to get her Social Security card to find a job and help out her parents. Her parents then told her she was undocumented, as was her entire family. When Yesenia and Julian met, she disclosed her status to him. He was not very concerned, as he had no idea how complicated the adjustment process would be. They married and within three years had a son and a daughter. Yesenia had attended college but did not pursue a master's degree, as she did not qualify for financial aid, and they were saving to build a home. Moreover, Yesenia did not want her husband to pay for her education, as they had many bills and she would not be able to work, given her undocumented status, even if she obtained more advanced degrees. The couple had been waiting with anticipation for the passage of the Dream Act, which would have granted legal status to persons like Yesenia, who had been brought to the United States as children by their parents. However, as consideration of passage of the Dream Act was delayed, the couple decided to proceed with adjusting her status. When the Dream Act failed to pass, Julian and Yesenia sought legal counsel and began the adjustment process.

Yesenia had to leave for Mexico and took the children with her, because they were too small for Julian to take care of. Neither expected the separation would be long. However, in the first interview, Yesenia was denied a pardon, despite the fact that she did not voluntarily come to the United States and instead was brought as a baby. She was told she would not be able to reenter the United States for ten years. Her husband was devastated. His wife had to travel to Michoacán to live with distant relatives, as her entire family had been in the United States for years. Julian was distraught.

He had worked in construction as a young man and had started his own construction company with his brothers. He had built his family a home where they lived for a few months before his family had to leave. He could not bear to be in the house without his wife and children and at times slept in the car or in his office. He did not tell his brothers or parents that he was not staying at his house, as he did not want to appear weak. He sought a new attorney, who reapplied for a pardon. Following his attorney's advice, Julian consulted me for an evaluation of extreme hardship.

When I met Julian, his wife had been in Mexico for two years. Julian was clinically depressed. He also had untreated PTSD as a result of his military service. Moreover, he was outraged. "I risked my life for this country, my country," he stated. "My wife did nothing wrong. She was a baby when she came to the United States. Why are my children being punished? They are Americans, as I am; why am I being punished? What kind of country is this that separates families?" Julian was suicidal and had significant homicidal ideation. He had fantasies of "going postal" and threatened that if his wife was not granted residency, he might do something crazy.

Julian worked because his family's subsistence depended on it. However, his brother stepped in and worked with him and for him on the days Julian could not get out of bed. He had lost weight and was irritable and anxious. Indeed, Julian met criteria for extreme hardship, as he had faced economic pressures, developed hypertension, and experienced severe psychiatric distress. As a third-generation Chicano, Julian did not think of himself as Mexican. He was American. The separation from his family, the erosion of his faith in his country, the United States, and the prejudiced attitudes he encountered during the legal process made him bitter.

Despite having a stable income and having attained economic success, as well as having access to health care, Julian had not sought treatment for his symptoms of depression and anxiety prior to and after his wife's departure. "Going to a shrink was not something one did," he stated. He was a man; he was supposed to handle things on his own. He was embarrassed that he cried for a long time in my presence; he apologized and was comforted by my telling him that being able to let his pain out made him a stronger man and could well lower his blood pressure.

Julian was at extreme risk when we met—he was suicidal, homicidal, and on the verge of a breakdown. He had untreated PTSD from the Gulf War, a preexisting condition, which was exacerbated by his wife's departure to Mexico. I insisted that his feelings and reactions were normal, given the situation. He was not crazy, but he needed support. He agreed to seek treatment—privately, however. He did not want to go to the VA hospital, as he was disillusioned by the US government and its institutions.

■ Heteronormativity, Homophobia, Transphobia, and Sexuality

Chicano gay, bisexual, and transgendered men encounter multiple challenges in their identity development (as discussed in chapter 2), which can impact their mental health in adulthood. As Richard A. Rodriguez (2004) has indicated, the growing literature on gay and bisexual men of color focuses on the "pull" to choose either a racial/ethnic or a sexual identity. Such a forced choice is untenable and unjust, and therefore stressful. Integration of one's multiple identities and finding validation in one's various communities are essential aspects of finding balance and mental health. A great deal of the literature on GBT Latinos and Chicanos explores the relationship between sexuality and problem behaviors that increase health risk—substance abuse and unprotected sex (see Carballo-Dieguez 1989; Diaz 1998; Diaz et al. 1999; Morales 1990); Rodriguez 2004) (see chapter 5 for further elaboration).

Existing studies indicate that marginalization and lack of a supportive family and/or community contribute to depression, anxiety, and high-risk behaviors among gay Latinos and Chicanos (Rodriguez 2004; Trujillo 1997). These scholars argue for the need to develop treatment approaches and interventions that counter heteronormativity and are attuned to the culture and experience of GBT Latinos. Limited information still exists, however, to guide the treatment of mental health needs of gay Chicanos (see Almaguer 1993).

■ Vignette #14: Finding balance: To be a man and Chicano and Queer

Juan was twenty-one and a sophomore in college when we first met. He was referred to therapy by his college counselor, a gay white male, who felt that Juan's issues with his sexuality might be better understood by a Latino therapist. He referred Juan to me as I was the only Latino therapist he knew. Juan was a second-generation Chicano, raised in a rural community of Central California by a traditional immigrant family with strong Christian values. As he was the only son in a family of five children, Juan held a privileged position within the family. His parents had sacrificed to put him through school. Juan struggled academically in high school as he became increasingly aware of his homosexuality. He tried to hide it from his family and became very depressed. His high school counselor was supportive but did not have much experience working with gay youth. Juan felt supported by her but not understood. Juan attended the local junior college and worked part-time. He began to date girls to appease his parents but secretly dated men. He was very anxious about being found out.

When he transferred to a university a hundred miles from home, he began to identify as bisexual and found a supportive college community of gay Latinos. Juan indicated that he was shocked that Chicanos could be openly gay and not be afraid of retaliation from the larger Latino community. He continued to struggle with depression as he found himself living a "double life." He was the dutiful Christian son when he went to visit his parents, and the sometimes outspoken Queer-identified Chicano on the campus.

As his grades continued to suffer, largely due to his activism and need to work, he developed severe anxiety and sought treatment at the counseling center. Juan found it difficult to connect with his therapist; Juan felt his therapist wanted him to come out to his family to demonstrate pride in his sexuality and to be more authentic in his sexual experiences. Juan did not see the need to mortify his parents and potentially lose the love and support of his family.

Early in our therapeutic relationship, we discussed his comfort level working with a Latina instead of a gay Chicano therapist. He was comfortable with the referral, so we proceeded to work together. We explored Juan's multiple identities and the stress of negotiating not only his sexuality but his biculturality and growing ideological separation from his parents. He struggled with the idea of being a sinner (according to his parents' views) and the damnation of homosexuals preached by his church minister. He was a man of faith but could not embrace his parents' idea of Christianity. For Juan, coming to terms with his multiple identities and embracing his sexuality meant losing aspects of his identity. We worked on transforming the narrative of loss to one of inclusiveness or change. Drawing on the work of Gloria Anzaldúa (1987) and other Chicana/o Queer theorists (Almaguer 1993; Gaspar de Alba 2003a; Perez 2003), we explored the meaning of a Queer/Chicano identity.

As we explored the roots of his anxiety—fear of loss of his family and religious community, rejection from his parents, shame, and greater visibility—Juan recognized his inner strength and sought to make community with others who embraced a similar identity. Over time, Juan began to come out to his sisters, who were mostly supportive, and ultimately to his mother. His mother begged him not to tell his father; she feared the news would kill him, and she promised to pray for her son until Juan changed. However, she did not withdraw her love, as Juan had feared. Juan came to accept that his family would struggle with his sexuality and that this was an existential reality he would have to face until he felt ready to tell his father.

The psychological, emotional, and spiritual pain Chicano men experience as a result of microaggressions, discrimination, marginalization, and daily indignities (Franklin 2004) may manifest as aggression, stoicism, hardness, coldness, disinterest, substance abuse, and violence toward the self and others. What lie beneath the surface may be diseases of the tonal—the spirit has been injured, the soul has been wounded. From a western perspective we can understand the distress as depression, anxiety, somatization, substance abuse, and anxiety disorders such as panic attacks, phobias, or PTSD. Nevertheless, it is critical to understand the mental health of Chicano men contextually to reduce the barriers to treatment and, once they are in treatment, to offer culturally responsive, respectful services that both honor their dignity and challenge the problematic behaviors (Flores-Ortiz, Esteban, and Carrillo 1994).

■ Summary

A number of creative approaches to help Chicano men find balance through men's circles, drumming circles, and individual, group, and family therapy approaches have been pioneered by Carrillo and Zarza (2008), Tello (2008), and Flores-Ortiz, Esteban, and Carrillo (1994), among others. These treatment approaches are rooted in pre-Columbian values of harmony and healing in community and are informed as well by biomedical findings, particularly about the role of attachment in IPV and the sequelae of trauma to the brain, which can result in the self-regulation problems associated with addiction, depression, and violence (Ziegler 2002).

Community-based programs and national organizations have documented the need for compassionate approaches to male aggression (see the National Compadres Network, for example) and implemented culturally attuned programs (Instituto Familiar de la Raza, in San Francisco, including La Cultura Cura Youth Program, which offers alternatives to violence and incarceration, and Si a la Vida, which addresses the physical and mental health needs of GBT Chicanos; and Clínica de la Raza, in Oakland, California, which offers mental health services). However, as stated in chapter 2, prevention is key to maintaining balance. Likewise, strengthening the psyche and soul of Chicanos by and in the family is critical to reduce the impact of racism, classism, homophobia, and all forms of suffering and of soul wounding.

■ Discussion Questions

1. What factors contribute to a greater incidence of depression and substance abuse among second- and third-generation Chicanos?

2. What is the role of gender in the experience and manifestation of soul wounding among Chicanos?

3. How can families support their sons to become hombres nobles?

4. How would you describe the characteristics of an ideal Chicano?

■ Suggested Readings

Arévalo, Sandra P., Laia Bécares, and Hortencia Amaro. "Health of Incarcerated Latino Men." In *Health Issues in Latino Males,* ed. Marilyn Aguirre-Molina, Luisa N. Borrell, and William Vega, 139–57. New Brunswick, NJ: Rutgers University Press, 2010.

Carrillo, Ricardo, and Jerry Tello, eds. *Family Violence and Men of Color: Healing the Wounded Male Spirit.* 2nd ed. New York: Springer, 2008.

de la Torre, Adela, Rosa Gomez-Camacho, and Alexis Alvarez. "Making the Case for Health Hardship: Examining the Mexican Health Care System in Cancellation of Removal Proceedings." *Georgetown Immigration Law Journal* 25, no. 1 (2010): 93–116.

Franklin, Anderson J. *From Brotherhood to Manhood: How Black Men Rescue Their Relationships and Dreams from the Invisibility Syndrome*. New York: Wiley, 2004.

Gil, Andres, and William Vega. "Alcohol, Tobacco and Other Drugs." In Aguirre-Molina, Borrell, and Vega, *Health Issues in Latino Males,* 99–122. New Brunswick, NJ: Rutgers University Press, 2010.

Instituto Familiar de La Raza. http://www.ifrsf.org.

The National Compadres Network. http://www.nationalcompadresnetwork.com.

Perilla, Julia. L., Caroline A. Lippy, Alvina Rosales, and Josephine V. Serrata. "Domestic violence prevalence: Philosophical, methodological, and cultural considerations." In *Violence against Women and Children: Consensus, Critical Analyses, and Emergent Priorities*. Vol. 1, *Mapping the Terrain*. Washington, DC: APA. (in press).

Perilla, Julia L., Josephine V. Serrata, Joanna Weinberg, and Caroline A. Lippy. "Integrating Women's Voices and Theory: A Comprehensive Domestic Violence Intervention for Latinas." *Women and Therapy* 35, nos. 1–2 (2012): 93–105.

Poe-Yamagata, Eileen, and Madeline Wardes Noya. "Race Disparities in the Juvenile Justice System." In *Race, Culture, Psychology, and Law,* ed. Kimberly Holt Barrett and William H. George, 311–345. Thousand Oaks, CA: Sage, 2005.

Polo, Antonio, and Margarita Alegria. "Psychiatric Disorders and Mental Health Service Use among Latino Men in the United States." In Aguirre-Molina, Borrell, and Vega, *Health Issues in Latino Males,* 183–211.

Sue, Derald W. *Microaggressions in Everyday Life: Race, Gender, and Sexual Orientation*. New York: John Wiley and Sons, 2010.

Villa, Velentine V., Nancy Harada, and Anh-Luu Huynh-Hohnbaum. "The Causes and Consequences of Poor Health among Latino Vietnam Veterans: Parallels for Latino Veterans of the War in Iraq." In Aguirre-Molina, Borrell, and Vega, *Health Issues in Latino Males,* 123–38.

5

Sexualities

Sexuality encompasses an individual's sex, gender identity and expression, and sexual orientation (American Psychological Association 2010). How a person comes of age sexually in terms of these factors is greatly influenced by his or her cultural upbringing. As discussed in earlier chapters, Latino men and women often receive different messages and rules about sexuality and sexual expression. From childhood, gender and sexuality are interconnected, such that girls tend to receive stronger pronouncements about modesty, virginity, and proper conduct than do boys (Zavella 1997). Patricia Zavella's 2003 study of Mexicanas and Chicanas in Santa Cruz, California, highlights the impact of such messages on women's adult sexuality and sexual behavior. She found that despite nativity, both immigrant and US-born Mexican-origin women often were shamed by their parents, particularly their mothers, for their sexual inquisitiveness. Parents rarely spoke to them about sex or directly expressed their expectations about "proper conduct." Often the messages were indirect and conveyed through innuendo and *moralejas,* stories about the negative outcomes of undesired behaviors. Furthermore, the women interviewed received strong messages of what Caridad Souza (2001) refers to as "that puta thing that just doesn't go away." "Specific gender and gender ideologies governed my behavior as a young girl and adolescent in this community. The label *puta* (whore) was used in this Latino community for girls and young women to uphold the rigid lines of sexual propriety" (Souza 2001, 119).

What does it mean to be a woman, to be a man in contemporary Mexican/ Chicano families? How do stereotyping and cultural ideals influence the embodiment of gender and sexuality among Mexican/Chicano men and women? What is the impact of such "rigid lines of sexual propriety" on the emotional, psychological, and physical well-being of Chicanas? How does the freedom to explore and come to terms with their sexuality influence Chicanos' well-being? This chapter explores these questions and highlights the limited research available on these topics.

■ Problematizing Latina/o Sexuality

Most of the social and psychological literature on Latina sexuality focuses on their reproductive patterns, specifically the high rates of teen pregnancy and the high fertility of Mexican and Mexican-origin women. Therefore, Chicana sexuality is cast as intrinsically problematic and invariably is associated with reproductive health issues (Biggs et al. 2010). Teen pregnancy is indeed an important public health concern, given the association of early pregnancy with poverty and multiple health disparities, including increased risk for substance use and abuse by adolescent sons of single-parenting women who were teen mothers (Gil and Vega 2010). Moreover, while Latina teen pregnancy rates decreased slightly in the past decade, Latina (and especially Chicana) teen pregnancy rates remain the highest of all ethnic groups. According to the National Campaign to Prevent Teen Pregnancy (2006, cited in Biggs et al. 2010), 51 percent of Latinas will have at least one pregnancy during their adolescence, and one in five sexually active Latino adolescent males will cause a pregnancy.

Furthermore, the age of first sexual activity has become younger among Latino and Latina teens, with boys reporting sixteen and a half as the average age for first intercourse. However, 11 percent of Latino boys reported having sex prior to age thirteen (Aguirre-Molina and Betancourt 2010). Biggs and colleagues also found that most Latino males described their first sexual experience as desired; Latinas did not. For many young women, the first sexual encounter is one where they often feel coerced by their boyfriends or partners (Biggs et al. 2010; Flores 2006).

The sexual behavior of Latina/os also becomes a public health concern due to their low rates of contraceptive use, in particular the low frequency of condom use by males during their first intercourse, which is predictive of later condom use (Biggs et al. 2010). Likewise, the risk of sexually transmitted infections (STIs), and HIV/AIDS in particular, is associated with lack of condom use. While adolescent Latino HIV/AIDS data are limited, the disproportionate rates of HIV infection among Latinos calls for increased education regarding reproductive health among the youth. Existing HIV/AIDS data indicate that HIV transmission patterns vary by national origin, birthplace, and geographic location. US-born Latinos account for 41 percent of the estimated AIDS cases among this population; those born in Puerto Rico and Mexico each constitute 22 percent of cases. The majority of Latinos living with AIDS reside in California, New York, and Puerto Rico (Biggs et al. 2010).

The sexual behaviors of Latinas and Latinos are associated with a number of risk factors, in particular lack of family cohesion, limited communication about sexuality, poverty, family disintegration, and lack of access to reproductive health education and services. However, adherence to cultural practices, parental education beyond high school, and communication about sexuality with parents emerge as important protective factors (Ayala 2006; Biggs et al. 2010). As with other issues affecting Chicano mental health, a combination of structural, community, and family factors influence attitudes about sexuality and sexual behaviors.

■ Coming-of-Age Rituals

The *quinceañera* or *quince,* the coming-of-age ritual practiced among many Chicano families, has been studied extensively by anthropologists, sociologists, and Chicano scholars and critiqued by Chicana feminists (see Cantu and Najera-Ramirez 2002; Davalos 1997). As a ritual the quince is meant to acknowledge a girl's coming of age—the beginning of her adulthood—as well as her purity, as exemplified by her wearing white. Some refer to it as a wedding rehearsal (Zavella 2003). In traditional Mexican culture, among the wealthier classes the quince also served as an announcement to potential suitors that the girl was available for marriage. For contemporary Chicano families, particularly those who have not held strong cultural ties to Mexico, the ritual may be practiced less frequently and may have more of a social than a religious/cultural meaning.

The importance of the ritual varies by nativity, class, and level of acculturation. Nevertheless, the anticipation of a girl's coming of age often is fraught with anxiety for parents and girls alike. Elena, a fourteen-year-old girl, viewed it this way:

> My parents want to have a big *pachanga* (party) and have spent way too much money on this event. I really do not want to have it. I have had to learn the waltz, which is ridiculous to me. The waltz has nothing to do with my *cultura*. I also feel a lot of guilt, because the white dress signifies virginity, and I am no longer a virgin. Of course, my parents do not know that. I have to go to Mass, and I have to confess, and I don't really feel like telling the priest about my sexual activities. I don't trust he will keep it a secret, as he knows my parents.

Elena was distressed by this situation; thus, she spoke to her high school counselor about it. Elena also was upset that her older brother did not have to go through what she termed "the circus" and was free to date. Elena had been seeing her boyfriend secretly and was not using condoms; she was afraid her mother would find them, since her mother regularly searched her room, backpack, and purse. Elena feared that if her parents found out about her sexual activity, she would fall from the pedestal and become a puta in her family's eyes. She believed that even her brother would turn against her if he found out that she was sexually active. In this family, standards of purity were upheld for the daughters, but not the sons.

While contemporary Chicano males do not have culturally sanctioned rituals of coming of age as did indigenous men, they are often placed in the position of being the guardians of their sisters' virtue. Also, they often hold a double standard, as did Sergio (chapter 4), who was sexually unfaithful to his partner but demanded her loyalty and already worried about his young daughter's adolescence, even though it was ten years away. He was socializing his son to protect his sister from men like himself.

■ Dealing with Contradictions

Chicanas often describe their coming of age as sexual beings as experiences fraught with contradictions. As women of color, they are frequently objectified as exotic, lascivious, and hot. They are simultaneously stereotyped as barefoot, pregnant, dark, and low-class. Their families may impose ideals of purity and virginity that may be difficult (or undesirable) for young women to attain, since they are bombarded with sexual images in the media. Stereotyped images of how a Latina is supposed to be can have a deleterious impact on self-image and self-esteem and can contribute to unhealthy behaviors, such as dieting and disordered eating (Chamorro and Flores-Ortiz 2000).

A number of studies find that Chicana adolescents experience stress as a result of voiced and unvoiced parental expectations about their sexuality. Young women often express a desire for their parents to discuss these issues openly (Ayala 2012; Flores 2006). The lack of "talking about sex" (Zavella 2003), along with rigid gender socialization, increases the chances for Chicanas to engage in high-risk practices that can affect their health as a result of sexually transmitted infections and diseases, such as cervical cancer and HIV/AIDS (Castañeda 2000).

Lack of information about sex and birth control methods, or reluctance to use them for fear of being found out, contributes to the high pregnancy rate among Latinas, especially Chicanas (Flores 2006). Moreover, Zavella (2003) found that young adult and more mature Chicanas and Mexicans used particular metaphors to describe their experience of sexuality and sexual exploration—playing with fire, hot, passionate, boiling, a fire that was difficult to control (342). As adolescents the women feared not being in control of their sexuality or being controlled by desire. These metaphors reflect in part the objectification and stereotyping Chicanas encounter in their everyday experience. They also reflect the perception of sexuality as dangerous and potentially hurtful to women.

While young Latinas and Chicanas are objectified, middle-aged Chicanas complain about becoming invisible. "There seems to be an assumption that I am sexless since I became a grandmother," stated Ofelia, a fifty-seven-year-old, recently divorced, second-generation Chicana. "My children expect me to be an abuelita (grandmother), in the style of my own mother, who sacrificed her sexuality first for the children and then for the grandchildren. My son told me that if I start dating, he will have to go into therapy." She offered to help pay for it.

Chicanas at midlife often struggle with balancing obligations toward parents and children and creating a space for their own desires, including sexual expression and the enjoyment of sex without concerns about reproduction (Flores-Ortiz 1997b). Cultural nicknames spouses use for each other such as *viejo/a* (old man/woman) as terms of endearment do not convey messages of sexual vibrancy. Chicanas in my practice often complain that when they finally arrive at a point in life where they can be more sexually free, our youth-oriented culture renders them less attractive. These women also struggle with the expectations of age-appropriate propriety, which they internalized when younger. While generational, age, and class differences do exist in women's relationships to their sexuality; women invariably encounter "that puta thing," and preoccupation about how others perceive them can create stress.

Likewise, cultural expectations that women should be cared for by men are stressful for women who do not have male partners due to divorce or separation. Julieta, a forty-seven-year-old, second-generation Chicana, was told by her older brothers that she should move in with her parents after her husband left her. She should not live alone. "It is not safe for a woman to live alone," they stated. While she appreciated their concern, she had no intention of returning to her parents' home; however, she felt conflicted between her own desire for continued independence and the traditional cultural script.

Women's bodies at times become the battleground of conflicting desires and expectations or the map where violence is recorded (Flores 2003). Many adult Chicanas in my clinical practice experienced shaming from their parents, as attention was called to their bodies (being too thin or too fat, having large breasts or wide hips, or being "thick") while being told to cover it up. Others discussed how women in their families were taught to be "sexy good girls" who could show but not allow a touch, lest men would not respect them. *"Hay que anunciar para vender; pero si das a probar, nadie va te lo va a comprar"* (You have to advertise to sell; but if you give free samples, no one will buy). This was a saying many of my Chicana clients heard while growing up. They came to see their bodies as commodities to be exchanged for financial security. Few recalled being taught to appreciate or care for their bodies for their own enjoyment.

The focus on women's sexuality as a commodity has historical roots from the time of the conquest. Pre-Columbian women in the Americas were taught to cherish their bodies and their own rights over themselves; sexuality often was connected directly to spirit and heart (Castillo 1995). The rape of indigenous women and the birth of the mestizo in many instances were used against women, as if they had willingly given themselves to the conqueror rather than being the victims of rape and genocide. The rape of indigenous women was recast as an example of women's treachery. The raped indigenous woman was blamed for the conquest and the downfall of Mexico. This historical trauma has impacted the relationship of men and women over generations. The shame of the conquest and the original rape of indigenous women has been passed down to *las hijas de Malinche*.[1]

As a result, men often distrust women, since they are socialized to believe that women are by nature manipulative and deceitful. Many men also are socialized to desire and fear a woman's sexuality and therefore are encouraged to contain and control it, presumably for her own good. Such cultural scripts promote secrecy and silence regarding sexuality. Chicanos also face stereotyped perceptions of their sexuality (Sluzki 1976).

Carlos Sluzki (1976) addressed the psychological impact on Latino men of having to uphold "the myth of the Latin lover." This myth, reified by Hollywood and Mexican cinema, positions men as violent sexual perpetrators or charming Don Juans who can sweep women off their feet with a simple gaze. Denise Chávez (2001), in her novel *Loving Pedro Infante,* describes the prototype of the Mexican macho, as embodied by movie icon Pedro Infante.

> He was incredibly handsome in that way only Mejicanos can be. I can't explain this to you, only a Mejicana or an intuitive gringa knows what I mean. The handsomeness and sexiness come on you slowly and then hit you between the eyes. The more you contemplate a man like Pedro, observe his mannerisms, stare into his eyes, delight in his unique smile and strong arms, trim waist and good legs, and watch how gentle and self-assured he is with people of all ages, and see how much they love him, you will begin to understand a little of what Pedro Infante means to me . . . (31)

Contemporary Mexican icons reflect more of a metrosexual image, such as Gabriel Garcia Bernal, who is now considered to embody the Mexican masculine ideal. Interestingly, Gabriel Garcia Bernal is light-skinned and European-looking. If he is indeed the embodiment of the Mexican masculine ideal, what is the message to more indigenous-looking men? Julian, a twenty-six-year-old, second-generation, heterosexual Chicano engineer, stated:

> When I was a teenager I could not live up to the ideal of attractiveness I was bombarded with. I did not look like Brad Pitt. I am short, dark, and solid. I look like my bracero grandfather, and my gardener dad. Those were my models. I was not popular. That actually helped me. I did not chase girls, I chased calculus. But as an adult I still have to contend with women's expectations of what a Mexican man or Chicano is supposed to be.

While Julian did not have self-esteem problems regarding his looks, he did feel at times objectified and offended by the expectations of sexual prowess held by some of the women he dated. "It hurts me, you know. Sometimes women expect me to be some hot Latin lover, romantic, athletic in bed. I am just a regular guy. I understand how women feel at times, now, I think. Women (white women, I mean) meet me and begin to talk about how I am probably a good dancer and good lover. It is a total turn-off."

These microagressions wounded Julian. He joked that he was going to let his mother find him a wife so he would not have to go through the hassle of courtship and thus avoid the way in which he felt sexualized and objectified by some women.

Men also experience silence regarding sexuality in their upbringing. Few of the Chicano students, research participants, and male clients I have had in over thirty years of professional life had conversations about sex and sexuality with their fathers, other adult males, or their mothers. An exception seemed to occur among Chicano men who grew up with single mothers. Ernesto, a twenty-two-year-old college student, recounted how his mother sat him down when he was thirteen and talked to him about being a responsible man. She talked to him about values and expectations, as well as the mistakes she had made in her life.

> She straight out told me, "Son, you are going to feel things in your body that may be strange, unfamiliar, and even pleasurable. As you get older you are going to want to have sex. Talk to me about it, before, you know. We can buy condoms for you. I don't want you to get any girl in trouble. You need to study so you won't have a hard life." I was, like, wow, my mom is pretty cool—I was not embarrassed or anything at the time. That made it easy for me to talk to her about sex later on when I needed to.

Citing the Youth Risk Surveillance data, which compared Latino, African American, and European American teens, Biggs and colleagues (2010) reported that Latino boys were the group least likely to discuss sexuality or condom use with their parents. Those who did tended to have fathers with more education.

The majority of my Chicano students, however, learned about sex from peers or older male family members who conveyed messages that sexual desire was normal and that men had the right to engage in sexual activity without commitment. The men also were told about good and bad women. Good women were to be wives; the others were to be used for sexual experimentation, to get experience. Jorge was told, as were several other men, that mothers, sisters, and female relatives were to be respected. He was not to lay a hand on them. However, all other women were "fair game." Jorge was conflicted about the messages he received. It did not seem fair to him that he should use women in this way. But he kept his opinions to himself. He did not want to be accused of being gay—*joto*—which is how his male relatives referred to young men who were virgins.

Of particular concern to Biggs and colleagues was the finding that both male and female Latino teens considered teen pregnancy a positive event, even if unplanned. For some teens, reproduction fills a void and offers them the chance to feel important and be needed. The high value of maternity among some Latinos may create a strong connection between reproduction and sexuality for teens. Most studies find that teen pregnancy is more likely to occur among academically disengaged, US-born adolescents who are growing up in single-parent and low-income households. These youth face a number of health disparities, in particular lack of sex education and limited information about family planning (Biggs et al. 2010). Clearly, both structural factors and family characteristics contribute to high-risk sexual behaviors, which threaten the psychological well-being of Chicana/os. Likewise, throughout their lives, Chicana/os encounter contradictive and disparaging messages about their sexuality and ethnicity that can wound their hearts and spirits.

◼ Latino Gays and Lesbians

Implicit in the gender socialization of Chicanas and Chicanos is an expectation of heterosexuality. Lesbians in Zavella's (2003) study recounted how their parents never talked about sexuality, and if homosexuality was ever mentioned, it was in denigrating and pejorative terms. Carla Trujillo (1997, 2001) describes the challenges of coming to terms with her sexuality growing up in a working-class Chicano family. She discusses "the girls our mothers warned us about"—the tomboys who might become lesbians, and the promiscuous girls who would never find a good man to marry them. As Hardy and Laszloffy (2005) argue, such experiences of devaluation impact the self-esteem and emotional well-being of gay and lesbian youth and may lead to depression and even suicide.

Oliva Espin (1987, 2012), Vivienne Cass (1979), and Eduardo Morales (1990), among others, posit that unlike heterosexuals, gays and lesbians must contend with a unique psychological aspect of sexuality, the coming-out process. Moreover, as Espin (2012) argues, "sexuality is always multilayered and individual desire is never purely individual" (46). Heterosexuals do not need to announce their sexual orientation. It is assumed and celebrated, as it is through the ritual of the quinceañera. Moreover, coming out is not a one-time event; it is a lifelong process, which differs depending on the relationship: family, friends, coworkers, community/ies, etc. It involves a reoccurrence of the different stages of identity formation and potential reexperiencing of the conflicts these stages represent.

For Chicana/o gays and lesbians, coming out may be experienced as a form of cultural suicide—given the risk of family loss and community marginalization. As a result of the racism and discrimination Chicana/os routinely encounter, the support of family and community is essential for psychological survival (Rodriguez 2004). Often there are generational (and regional) differences in how Latino gays and lesbians come out (Espin 1987; Morales 1990). In more progressive and accepting communities, gay youth may have safe spaces and groups (in junior and senior high school, for example) and therefore, may be more prepared to be out when they go to college or enter the workforce. They also may have support to deal with the family crisis or possible rejection that may occur once there is a disclosure of their sexual orientation.

In communities, settings, or families that are intolerant, youth may be forced to hide their sexuality, as it would be unsafe to disclose it. Sexual identity formation in and of itself may be fraught with conflict, given the pervasive cultural messages of heteronormativity. The process of gay/lesbian identity formation is more complex for immigrants and individuals who are members of particular religious groups (Espin 1987). Latina/o gays and lesbians must face particular issues; already marginalized and othered as persons of color, they must confront another source of discrimination and marginalization based on their sexual orientation and expression. Often gay and lesbian Latinos and Chicanos feel they must choose between their cultural and their sexual community. As discussed in chapter 3, such forced untenable choices can result in feelings of devaluation, despair, depression, and ultimately suicide. The stress experienced as a result of devaluation may be managed in maladaptive ways, through the use of alcohol or drugs or unprotected sexual practices (see Diaz 1998). It can also be addressed in constructive ways if the youth and adults have family, peer, or community support.

An essential aspect of adolescent development is the integration of gender, ethnic, racial, and sexual identities. The majority of identity development models focus on one aspect of this process. There remains a lack of analysis of how young people make sense of their multiple identities and attain a sense of self that is as complex as their experience. Morales's (1990) model of sexual identity formation for Latino gays and lesbians incorporates the dual minority status of being gay and of color. He proposes a five-state model.[2] In the first state, there may be a denial of conflicts as individuals attempt to deny their sexuality or that their sexuality could be a source of crisis or conflict. In the second state, the conflict is between identifying as bisexual vs. gay or lesbian. The individual may be reluctant to claim a homosexual identity, may identify as bi, or simply deny that sexual identity is relevant. Juan, a twenty-eight-year-old, second-generation Chicano, asked, "Why do I have to label myself? That is a gay white thing. Besides, if I come out, my family will disown me and I will face even more discrimination than I do now as a result of being Chicano."

In the third state, there may be a conflict in allegiances—the individual is put in (or feels put in) the untenable position of choosing between an ethnic and sexual identity as a result of homophobia in the culture and racism in the gay/lesbian community. Subsequently, in the fourth state, there is a need to establish priorities in allegiances—the individual struggles with answering the complex question "Who am I?" and with deciding which identity is more salient within a particular context. Am I Chicana first or a lesbian first? Can I be both gay and Chicano in my community? In the final state, the focus is on integrating the various communities—the extent to which an individual can find support and acceptance within the communities to which she or he belongs will facilitate the process of coming out and integration (Almeida, Dolan-Del Vecchio and Parker 2007).

Espin (1987) and Morales (1990) note that special challenges for Latino gays and lesbians are presented by the multiple layers of oppression they face and the possible rejection by the family. Latino cultures, with the emphasis on reproduction and parenting, often will not consider normal an individual who does not marry someone of the opposite sex; families may tolerate a member's homosexuality but may not want anyone outside the immediate family to know, for fear of "*el que diran*" (what people will say). Thus, Latina/os may need to hide an essential aspect of their identity to remain connected to their family.

Acceptance of being both a Latina and a lesbian appears to become easier with age, as Espin (2012) found in her study of Latina lesbians who were mostly Cuban and Puerto Rican and who had attained professional status through education. For younger women, there were salient conflicts of loyalty and frustration with having to choose between equally important identities—their cultural and sexual identification—which some respondents saw as being the product of racism and homophobia (48).

Furthermore, coming out may jeopardize an individual's place in the family and the community. Thus, many Latinas and Latinos do not disclose their sexual orientation (Rodriguez 2004). Espin (2012) found that many of the Latina lesbians in her study felt the need to remain closeted because they feared that coming out would jeopardize "not only strong familial ties, but also the possibility of working for the betterment of the Latino community" (49), as they might be rejected because of their sexuality. To what extent these concerns exist among Chicana lesbians is not known.

Latino men may live dual lives, which can be stressful and are likely to contribute to high-risk behaviors, including alcohol and other drug misuse or abuse and unprotected sex (Diaz and Ayala 1999). In their studies of Latino gay men, Diaz and Ayala identified a number of contextual factors that increase high risk behavior. These authors postulated that among gay Latinos interpersonal experiences of racial discrimination lead to low self-esteem, a perception of diminished personal control, and fatalism regarding the inevitability of contracting HIV among gay Latinos. Furthermore, Diaz and colleagues (Ayala and Diaz 2001) posit that oppression, which is prevalent in the lives of Latino gay men, adds to the vulnerability produced by social class, which ultimately increases the risk to engage in unsafe sexual practices. Lack of social support, male sexual behaviors, and perception of an incompatibility between trust, love, intimacy, and condom use also contribute to high risk of HIV infection (Diaz and Ayala 1999).

Men who live dual lives are more likely to infect their female partners with HIV. The majority of HIV-positive Latinas (70 percent) were infected through sexual contact (Centers for Disease Control and Prevention 2008a). Clearly, the disparagement gay Latino and Chicano men experience can affect their health and that of the women with whom they have sexual relations.

Latina and Latino gays and lesbians are a minority within the European American gay community and may not be able to fully experience their multiple identities. This in turn can impact their emotional and spiritual well-being. Heterosexual Latinos may stereotype, discriminate, and otherwise render invisible Latino gays and lesbians as a function of heterosexual privilege, homophobia, or religious/cultural values. The end result of such soul wounding may be depression and/or substance abuse. A supportive social system is essential to counter family rejection and society devaluation when it occurs, in order to promote and maintain emotional, physical, and spiritual balance among LGBTQ Chicanos. Moreover, spirituality and religious beliefs, irrespective of their source, can be a source of support and emotional well-being for gay, lesbian, and bisexual individuals (Espin 2012).

■ Transgendered Chicana/os

Little information is available regarding the challenges encountered by trans-gendered Latina/os and Chicana/os (Nemoto, Operario, and Keatley 2005). As Anzaldúa (1987) has argued, queer Latinas and Latinos contest funda-mental cultural notions of sexuality; transgendered Latina/os must fight for the right to be human beings, along with challenging dual cultural construc-tions of gender and sexuality. As with other members of LGBTQ commu-nities, transgendered men and women must challenge cultural notions of fe/maleness and stereotypes about gender, and negotiate structural, cultural, and personal barriers to access needed health and mental health services.

In their studies of male-to-female (MtF) transgendered individuals of color in the San Francisco Bay Area, Nemoto and colleagues (2004, 2005) found "alarming levels of HIV, drug abuse and mental health need" (Nemoto et al. 2005, 6) among the women. Transgendered Latinas reported higher levels of depression, substance abuse and HIV risky behaviors when compared to African American and Pacific Islander transgendered women. Moreover, Latinas also experienced more barriers to obtaining health care, substance abuse treatment, housing, and social and mental health services. They also were dissatisfied with many of the service providers, who lacked knowledge about transgenderism sufficient to treat, guide, counsel, or sup-port them with respect to their complex needs. Furthermore, given the discrimination transgendered women encounter, they have limited work opportunities. As a result, sex work is often the only viable form of employ-ment. In turn, such work creates risk factors for substance abuse, as the women drink or use drugs to cope with the demeaning work and the vio-lence that often accompanies that profession (Nemoto et al. 2005). Perhaps as a result of the health disparities created by the structural barriers MtF transgendered women face, a large number of the Latinas in the sample obtained hormones from friends or from Mexico, where hormones can be purchased without prescription. Some Latinas also attempted to change their appearance by using silicone injections obtained from nonmedical sources, which increases the risk of infection and even death.

Nemoto and colleagues' findings are of concern; San Francisco City and County has specialized services for transgendered individuals and is known to be a city respectful of sexual diversity. Still, MtF transgendered individuals of color expressed dissatisfaction with existing health care services and significant need for additional social services. Their findings also point to the need to develop transgendered-specific services for people of color and better training for service providers. Transgendered Chicanas and Chicanos require compassionate and well-trained mental health providers who can address the psychological, social, cultural, and spiritual needs unique to their experience. The family also can play a central role in supporting transgendered Latina/os' search for physical, emotional, and spiritual wholeness.

■ Vignette #15: "I finally get to be who I have known I am"

John was sixteen and a high school sophomore when we met. I was invited to speak about Latino family issues to his school-based counseling group, which was facilitated by a former student of mine. John was third-generation. His grandfather had come to the United States as a young man; his parents were both born in the United States. John, who was named Juana at birth, stated that he always felt that he was in the wrong body. From the time he was in elementary school, he refused to wear dresses. His father could not understand John's behavior and became very frustrated with him. When the parents discussed their concerns with his pediatrician, they were referred to therapy.

To John's surprise, his grandfather emerged as his strongest ally when he disclosed to the therapist and the family that he wanted to undergo surgery to become a man. The therapist offered to work with the family to explore John's desire to have surgery. The parents refused to pay for the treatment unless the therapist worked to make "Juana normal." His grandfather articulated passionately and authoritatively that John had the right to be himself. He recounted his years of struggle to build a family in the United States. He was appalled that his son, witness to the multiple injustices faced by the family, would be so unjust with his own child. As the parents struggled to understand John's "confusion," the grandfather stated: "If he feels like a man, he is a man. Period, end of conversation." "Why do people in this country make things so complicated?" he added. After many sessions of heart-wrenching family therapy, John's parents offered to send out new birth announcements, if John so desired, after his surgeries were complete.

In this case the family's love for their child was stronger than their own notions of gender, sexuality, and normalcy. Not all queer or transgendered Chicana/os experience such levels of support. When family support is absent, the risk for mental health problems increases.

◼ Negotiating Cultural, Ethnic, and Sexual Identities

Many immigrant and second-generation Chicanos associate alternative lifestyles with the dominant European American culture and perceive children who do not adhere to traditional gender roles and behaviors as overacculturated or somehow lost to the culture of origin. Espin's essay notes how some Latina/os describe lesbianism as "an illness we catch from American women" (2012, 45). That is, some family members attribute their children's sexual/affectional orientation to acculturation to US culture. In such cases, family members and LGBTQ Chicana/os can experience psychological and emotional distress.

◼ Vignette #16: "What did I do wrong?"

Elliot, a third-generation, mixed-parentage man (his mother was Mexican and his father Anglo) sought couples therapy because his wife, Jennifer (European American), was distraught about their seventeen-year-old son Mark's disclosure that he might be gay. His son also identified with punk rock and dressed "punk." Furthermore, Jennifer was deeply religious and feared that Mark's lifestyle was satanic. Mark considered his parents ridiculous and reactionary, and his father to be whitewashed.

Mark had been interested in learning about his Mexican ancestry since childhood. His paternal grandmother had helped raise him and always spoke to him in Spanish, partly because she regretted not teaching Elliot about her language and culture. Mark was dark-skinned, unlike his mother and father. He was always "treated as a Mexican" at school. Therefore, he identified as such. Mark indicated that he was attracted to both males and females. However, he felt pressured by peers and the larger gay community in his public high school to choose being either gay or straight. Mark also was attracted to Latino punk music, which he perceived to be less racist and classist than white punk music.[3]

Elliot and Jennifer wondered what they had done wrong. Elliot stated that he "did not look Mexican"; therefore, he assimilated easily and, although he adored his mother, it was "easier" for him "to be white like his father." He had male and white privilege, he acknowledged. Jennifer had an uneasy relationship with her mother-in-law, whom she loved and respected. However, she was resentful of her and Mark's secret language (Spanish), which at times made her feel like an outsider. Jennifer stated that the grandmother had always wanted a daughter and that she had treated Mark "as a girl," which made him gay. Mark was incensed by her comment and was quite vocal, calling his mother racist, sexist, and ignorant.

Both parents felt that Mark, their only child, was rebelling against their religion and values. They felt that Mark was lost, as were many young people in their social circle. Mark argued that he was actually fulfilling his grandparents' American dream by fighting injustice and self-actualizing. The family remained polarized for some time. Mark continued in therapy, working on issues of sexuality because he did not want to conform to his parents' or the larger community's expectations that he declare his sexual orientation. Mark's grandmother saw his sexuality as the result of overacculturation; she blamed herself in part for not instilling more "Mexicanidad" (Mexicanness) in her son and grandson. She believed that being gay was a "white people's disease."

Arellano (2011) posits that punk culture provides a space for Latinos to negotiate their multiple identities, particularly when the youth have experienced familial and societal rejection due to their ethnicity, race, sexuality, or gender. Mark had the love and support of his family, despite their concerns and at times disapproval of his lifestyle. Eventually, they came to accept his identification with punk culture and his embracing of a Chicano bisexual identity.

■ Sexual Violence

The silences regarding sexuality prevalent in Chicano families are also reflected in the frequent denial of sexual violence when it occurs. As stated in earlier chapters, Chicanas experience high rates of intrafamily and domestic violence. Less is known about the sexual abuse of Chicano men. As with most men, reporting of such abuse is rare. In my own research (Flores 2006), Chicano college students disclosed having been fondled or molested by female relatives. In most instances, when they told their parents about the abuse, the experience was either minimized or not believed. The young men who were abused sexually as boys by male family members or acquaintances never disclosed the information. They carried the pain of the victimization quietly. They described feeling a rage inside that found no outlet. None of the young men had sought psychotherapy.[4]

Whether they had disclosed or not, the pervasive feeling experienced by these men was of guilt and shame. As is the case with women victims of sexual abuse, the men felt they should have done something to avoid or prevent the abuse, even if they were small children when it occurred. Joseph, a second-generation Chicano student disclosed that his grandfather had sodomized him for years. His first memory of the abuse was in Mexico, when the family had visited the grandparents. His grandfather was a well-known and respected businessman. He had a large study where he worked. He invited Joseph to see his books. Over a period of days, Joseph came to trust his grandfather. The study became their special place, where "Grandpa" gave him candy and told him stories. Within a few days, the "games" began. Grandpa would tickle and sit Joseph on his lap. One day he pulled down Joseph's pants and told him that he wanted to see if he had the family mark, because in his family males had big testicles. Then he pulled down his pants and showed Joseph his own sexual organs. Joseph remembers feeling uncomfortable and telling his grandfather he wanted to leave because he did not like the game. His grandfather grabbed him and forced his penis into Joseph's mouth. Joseph cried as he recounted the abuse that began in this manner. Joseph was sodomized daily after that. He became ill with nausea and high fever. His grandfather insisted on taking care of him. No one noticed the bruising or the rectal bleeding. Joseph became a sullen, withdrawn child. The abuse happened every summer, when Joseph was sent to visit his grandparents. As a young man he often had violent fantasies and questioned his sexuality. But he never told. He did not think anyone would believe him.

Julia had a similar story. She was abused by her uncle and, later, a friend of the family. She began cutting as an adolescent and struggled with eating disorders. When she first went to college, she experienced a date rape. While she obtained counseling after the rape, she did not disclose the childhood sexual victimization. She did not want that information to "be held against" her. Julia feared that a sexual abuse history would lead her counselor to think that she had "asked for it."

In my earlier work (Flores-Ortiz 1995, 1997a, 2003), I have discussed the spirit wounding and psychological trauma experienced by survivors of sexual violence. The healing of such trauma requires multiple interventions (van der Kolk 1994), because sexual violence affects the body, mind, heart, and spirit of those who are victimized. One aspect of healing that is most challenging is the reconnection of heart, mind, and body. Many sexual abuse survivors disconnect from their bodies; at times they despise their bodies because of the battlefield it became (Flores-Ortiz 1995, 1997a, 2003). When the body has been defiled, the individual feels dirty. A touch, a look, a sound, or a smell can trigger memories of the abuse and PTSD symptomatology. While some individuals are able to repress conscious memory of the abuse, the body remembers. Consequently, sexual dysfunction, avoidance of relationships, lack of pleasure in one's body, or increased high-risk sexual behaviors are common sequelae of sexual abuse and sexual violence (Flores 2003).

Many of my Chicana clients who are survivors of sexual violence carry deep spiritual wounds. The intergenerational trauma of the conquest is encoded in their psyche. When they experience sexual violence in their lives, they often connect to the histories of their female ancestors who endured the same. "Soy una más, soy una más," cried Nicole after a date rape. The police officer, who spoke no Spanish, did not understand. "I am one more, I am one more," she said. The officer believed she was referring to a possible serial rapist on campus. She later told me: "No one understands. Chicanas, we are connected by this history of misogyny. From the beginning we have been prey to men who try to control us, who sexualize us, who fight battles against other men on our bodies. No one understands what that feels like, to be so unprotected, to be such a prey."

The devastation experienced after sexual violence is reflected in depression, anxiety, panic, and susto. Men feel particularly powerless, because their gender socialization has convinced many that such things should not happen *to* men. Victor, a twenty-eight-year-old Chicano who was raped in juvenile hall at age fourteen, said: "We are the ones who should be *chingando,* not the ones who are *chingados.*" As a man, he believes, he should not experience forced sex; that is what men do—not have done to them. He experienced a brutal sexual attack after being sent to juvenile hall for tagging under a freeway. His working-class, single-parent mother could not afford a lawyer. He saw the rape as an act of violence, a ritual of initiation into the justice system. At that moment, he decided he would become a perpetrator, if need be, instead of a victim. Victor did not associate his subsequent substance abuse and depression with the violence he endured while detained as a juvenile.

■ Summary

A central aspect of mental health in both western and mestizo traditions is the integration of body, mind, and spirit. Acceptance and enjoyment of one's sexuality is an important component of physical and emotional well-being. For Chicanas and Chicanos such enjoyment is nuanced by cultural rules and dominant culture views on Chicanos as a people. As with other facets of mental health, family, community, and individual factors contribute to well-being or pain. Clearly, the entitlement to honor, respect, enjoy, and celebrate one's sexuality must be nurtured in the home. Likewise, healthy sexual identity development must be facilitated by the family and community. Respect for human integrity should include valuing human sexuality. The schools can play a key role in preventing sexual violence and promoting healthy sexuality; so can family and community activism to combat stereotyped and sexualized images of Chicanas and Chicanos, what Espin (2012) refers to as metanarratives that are rooted in and created by oppression. These metanarratives can be internalized and wound the soul, mind, and bodies of Chicanas and Chicanos.

■ Discussion Questions

1. What are some cultural protective factors regarding the sexual behavior of Chicana/o teens?

2. In what ways can families promote the healthy sexual identity development of their children?

3. What are the consequences of sexual violence on the lives of Chicana/os?

4. How can schools counter the microaggressions faced by Chicana/os regarding their gender, sexuality, and ethnicity?

5. Discuss the challenges faced by transgendered Latinas.

■ Notes

1. Malinche, or Malintzin, was a young princess who was given to Cortez as translator and interpreter. She became his lover and has been maligned as the symbolic mother of mestizos. To be a Malinche means to be treacherous, to betray one's man and culture. See Cordelia Candelaria, "La Malinche: Feminist Prototype," *Frontiers: A Journal of Women Studies* 5, no. 2 (1980):1–6,for a Chicana feminist reformulation of Malinche.

2. Unlike others, Morales does not use the term *stage*. He argues instead for the use of the term *state,* as he describes states of being in relation to one's sexuality, family, peers, and community. The focus is not on stages that are mastered, but on states that are experienced and possibly reexperienced over the lifetime.

3. For an excellent discussion of Latino punk culture, see Leticia Arellano's "A Subculture of a Culture: A Hermeneutic Study of the Latina/o-Chicana/o Punk Experience," doctoral dissertation. Wright Institute Graduate School of Psychology, Berkeley, 2011.

4. After the disclosure during the research project, the young men were referred to the campus counseling center. A few chose to seek private therapy. As a professor of psychology courses, I have heard numerous first-time disclosures over the years from both Chicano and Chicana students. Often the students begin to struggle academically as a result of PTSD symptomatology, yet they do not make a connection between their difficulties with concentration, the depression or anxiety they experience, and the childhood trauma of sexual abuse.

■ Suggested Readings

Almeida, Rhea "What Straight Therapists Can Do." *Family Magazine* 2, no. 4 (1997): 7–11.

Castañeda, Donna. "The Close Relationship Context and HIV Risk Reduction Behavior among Latinas/os." *Sex Roles* 42 (2000): 551–80.

Centers for Disease Control and Prevention. "HIV/AIDS among Hispanics/Latinos: Factsheet." Atlanta: Department of Health and Human Services, Centers for Disease Control and Prevention, 2005. http://www.cdc.gov/hiv/hispanics/resources/factsheets/hispanic.htm.

Centers for Disease Control and Prevention. "HIV/AIDS among Women: Factsheet." Atlanta: Department of Health and Human Services, Centers for Disease Control and Prevention, 2008a. http://www.cdc.gov/hiv/topics/women/resources/factsheets/women.htm.

Chamorro, Rebecca, and Yvette G. Flores-Ortiz. "Acculturation and Disordered Eating Patterns among Mexican American Women." *International Journal of Eating Disorders* 28, no. 1 (2000): 125–29. Reprinted in *Latina Health in the*

United States: A Public Health Reader, ed. Marilyn Aguirre-Molina and Carlos W. Molina. San Francisco: Jossey-Bass, 2003.

Diaz, Rafael M. *Latino Gay Men and AIDS: Culture, Sexuality and High-Risk Behavior.* New York: Routledge, 1998.

Espin, Oliva. "Cultural and Historical Influences on Sexuality in Hispanic/Latin Women: Implications for Therapy." In *Latina Realities: Essays on Healing, Migration and Sexuality,* ed. Oliva Espin, 83–96. Boulder, CO: Westview Press, 1987.

———. " . . . An Illness We Catch From American Women? The Multiple Identities of Latina Lesbians." *Women and Therapy* 35, nos. 1–2 (2012): 45–56.

———. "Issues of Identity in the Psychology of Latina Lesbians. In *Latina Realities: Essays on Healing, Migration and Sexuality,* ed. Oliva Espin, 97–110. Boulder, CO: Westview Press, 1987.

Flores, Yvette. "Rape." In *Latinas in the United States: An Historical Perspective,* ed. Virginia Sanchez Korrol, Vicki L. Ruiz, and Carlos Cruz, 611–13. Bloomington: Indiana University Press, 2005.

Flores-Ortiz, Yvette G. "The Broken Covenant: Incest in Latino Families." *Voces: A Journal of Chicana/Latina Studies* 1, no. 1 (1997): 48–70.

———. "Psychotherapy with Chicanas at Midlife: Cultural/Clinical Considerations." In *Racism in the Lives of Women,* ed. Jeanne Adelman and Gloria Enguídanos, 251–60. New York: Haworth Press, 1995.

———. "Re/membering the Body: Latina Testimonies of Social and Family Violence." In *Violence and the Body: Race, Gender, and the State,* ed. Arturo J. Aldama, 347–59. Bloomington: Indiana University Press, 2003.

———. "The Role of Cultural and Gender Values in Alcohol Use Patterns among Chicana/Latina High School and University Students: Implications for AIDS Prevention." *International Journal of Addictions* 29, no. 9 (1994): 1149–71.

Hurtado, Aida. *Voicing Chicana Feminisms: Young Women Speak Out on Sexuality and Identity.* New York: New York University Press, 2003.

Morales, Eduardo S. "Ethnic Minority Families and Minority Gays and Lesbians." In *Homosexuality and Family Relations,* ed. Frederick W. Bozett and Marvin D. Sussman, 272–97. New York: Haworth Press, 1990.

Nemoto, Tooru, Don Operario, and JoAnne Keatley. "Health and Social Services for Male-to-Female Transgender Persons of Color in San Francisco." *International Journal of Transgenderism* 8, nos. 2–3 (2005): 5–19.

Nemoto, Tooru, Don Operario, JoAnne Keatley, Lei Han, and Toho Soma. "HIV Risk Behaviors among Male-to-Female Transgender Persons of Color in San Francisco." *American Journal of Public Health* 94, no. 7 (2004): 1193–99.

Rodriguez, Richard. "Psychotherapy with Gay Chicanos." In *The Handbook of Chicano Psychology and Mental Health,* ed. Robert Velasquez, Leticia M. Arellano, and Brian McNeil, 193–214. Mahwah, NJ: Lawrence Erlbaum, 2004.

Souza, Caridad. "Esta risa no es de loca." In the Latina Feminist Group, *Telling to Live: Latina Feminist Testimonios,* 114–22. Durham, NC: Duke University Press, 2001.

Trujillo, Carla, ed. *Chicana Lesbians: The Girls Our Mothers Warned Us About.* Berkeley: Third Woman Press, 2001.

van der Kolk, Bessel A. "The Body Keeps the Score: Memory and the Evolving Psychobiology of Post-Traumatic Stress." *Harvard Review of Psychiatry* 1, no. 5 (1994): 253–65.

6

Mental Health and Aging

Finding Balance *en la Tercera Edad*

The degree of physical and mental health experienced by individuals in their "golden years"—defined in the United States as the age of retirement and in Latin America as "the third age"—is determined in large measure by the quality of life attained since childhood. Individuals who face health disparities are believed to be at greater risk for the onset of chronic illnesses in midlife, beginning in the decade of their forties. As chronic illnesses begin to take their toll in midlife, the quality of life is reduced. Chronic illnesses also contribute to shorter life expectancies for those who have lacked adequate health care. At present the leading causes of death for older US residents include heart disease, various cancers, respiratory illness (including pneumonia), and cerebrovascular diseases. While cognitive impairment may not directly result in death, it does contribute to a decreased quality of life for older adults; likewise, depression increases suicide risk for older persons (Alford and Espino 2010; Hinton et al. 2006).

The relative youthfulness of the US Latino population can obscure the fact that older Latinos represent the fastest-growing segment of those sixty-five and older in the United States and constitute the largest ethnic minority group among the aged. Moreover, 50 percent of these older Latinos are Mexican immigrants and first-generation children of immigrants (Alford and Espino 2010; Applewhite, Garcia Biggs, and Herrera 2010). It is estimated that by 2040, some 40 percent of the US population (about 15 million persons) over age sixty-five will be Latino.

A public health concern regarding the aging Mexican and Chicano population is its sociodemographic profile. This group in particular has faced a number of structural barriers—undereducation prior to migration, employment in low-skilled labor, limited access to health care services, and limited opportunities for acculturation post-migration—all of which increased their risk for living in poverty and contribute to the development of chronic illness. These factors contribute to the incidence of mental health problems as well, particularly mood and anxiety disorders. They are also risk factors for cognitive decline.

For Applewhite and colleagues (2010) successful aging and quality of life for Latinos are "largely described by interethnic and intraethnic differences and similarities based on cultural beliefs, values, traditions, behavioral patterns, life perspectives, socioeconomic status and health inequities" (235). This chapter examines the social and cultural context of Chicana/o elders and the limited information regarding their mental health status, in order to examine their aging process and quality of life.

■ The Health and Mental Health of Latino Elders

The Hispanic health paradox (Vega and Amaro 1994) remains evident with aging Latinos. Despite their higher levels of poverty and associated health disparities, their life expectancy and leading causes of death are not significantly different from those of European Americans with higher incomes and fewer disparities. However, Latinos—Mexican Americans in particular—do experience higher rates of diabetes and diabetes complications, as well as high rates of cognitive decline when compared to European Americans of the same age (Alford and Espino 2010). It is estimated that over 85 percent of Latinos have at least one chronic illness, which impairs their quality of life (Applewhite, Garcia Biggs, and Herrera 2010). These health problems can result in significant disability and increased depression among Chicanas and Chicanos.

Despite greater longevity when compared to European Americans and other ethnic minority groups, Latinos do not enjoy a comparable quality of life in their *tercera edad* when compared to their non-Latino peers (Applewhite, Garcia Biggs, and Herrera 2010). Using data from the Hispanic Established Populations for the Epidemiological Study of the Elderly (EPESE), Alford and Espino (2010) reviewed the structural barriers contributing to health decline among older Chicanos. In the EPESE study, 3,050 Mexican Americans were interviewed regarding their health; their information was then verified by medical records. There were similarities in the demographic profiles of Chicanas and Chicanos in the sample. Both males and females averaged 73 years in age. More than half were born in the United States, 55.2 percent of the men and 56.5 percent of the women. Despite nativity, the majority preferred to be interviewed in Spanish

(76.7 percent of the men and 78.7 percent of the women). The majority (82.0 percent for the men and 84.7 percent of the women) reported eight years of schooling or less. Most of the males and females reported incomes of less than $20,000 a year; 63.1 percent of the women and 50.6 percent of the men reported an annual income of $9,999 or less.

Notwithstanding a similar demographic profile, the authors found significant gender differences regarding overall health and living situation. More than twice as many women than men lived alone (34.1 percent and 16.6 percent respectively), suggesting that women are more likely than men to lose the extended family and spousal support that is normative in Latino cultures. This may contribute to their relative poverty and greater dissatisfaction with their overall health and higher levels of depression than were reported by the men.

An examination of chronic diseases by gender found some important differences between Chicanos and Chicanas; women had higher rates of diabetes, stroke and cancer. In addition, more women than men had hypertension (48.8 percent and 34.7 percent respectively) and arthritis (41.2 percent and 27.7 percent respectively). More women than men were likely to be obese. Chicano elders were more likely to be overweight than obese, which partly explains the larger percentage of women with diabetes in the sample. In fact, 66.9 percent of the women in the EPESE sample had diabetes, whereas 43.1 percent of the men were affected by that chronic illness. As stated previously, diabetes results in severe physical and psychological disability among the aged.

With regards to mental disorders, more men (12.6 percent) than women had a mental disorder (9.8 percent). However, more women than men had clinical levels of depression (28.7 percent and 17.2 percent respectively). Moreover, 38.8 percent of the women and 36.7 percent of the men experienced some level of cognitive decline. In addition, women manifested greater rates of depression or impairment (42.5 percent of the women and 38.2 percent of the men) or depression *and* impairment (12.5 percent and 7.9 percent respectively). A related finding is that men had slightly higher levels of self-esteem than women (4.69 percent and 4.61 percent respectively), although it was low overall and more men described being very or completely satisfied with their life (85.4 percent) than did women (81.7 percent). Of note is that despite their overall poor health and low socioeconomic status, most Chicana/os interviewed reported high life satisfaction.

The high rates of depression, particularly among Chicanas, are of concern, as is the cognitive decline associated with normal aging as well as dementing disorders. The EPESE study found that rates of cognitive impairment were influenced by age, education, literacy, language of interview, and marital and immigrant status. Thus, immigrants, Spanish-speakers, and those with low literacy and low education attainment showed greater degrees of impairment than younger, US-born, and economically more advantaged elders (Alford and Espino 2010). Gender was not a significant factor; however, males had a higher mortality rate in follow-up interviews eight years after the original EPESE data were collected; 35.9 percent of the men had died, compared to 26.6 percent of the women. Moreover, cognitive impairment, depression, or a combination of the two increased the risk of death for both men and women eight years after the original interviews.

Alford and Espino suggest that in addition to individual economic and health indicators, community factors such as segregated under-resourced communities and family characteristics, which can contribute to elder isolation, need to be considered to fully understand the impact of lifelong health disparities on Latino elders. Likewise, structural factors such as limited education, lack of social inclusion, and limited English skills all contribute to decreased quality of life and the burden of illness in the last decades of life. Of equal importance is the meaning of old age for Latinos, the values regarding elders, and the cultural changes that may diminish the influence and importance of the aged in contemporary Chicano families (see Flores 2008; Flores et al. 2009).

Studies of older Latinos find that this population associates well-being with physical, emotional, and spiritual health (*cuerpo, corazón, y alma*) and with good family and interpersonal relationships. Disharmony in any of these areas can contribute to stress, anxiety, depression, and cognitive decline, which in turn can diminish health and well-being (Beyene, Becker, and Mayen 2002).

■ Cultural Perceptions of Aging

In traditional Latino cultures *la tercera edad* is considered the stage of life when older men and women expect to reap the benefits of a life lived well. Among Latinos who hold traditional values, elders are to be respected, provided for, taken care of, and honored for their wisdom. If elders have followed traditional scripts, they married and had children. They will be blessed with grandchildren, and their adult children will provide financial and emotional support. Caregiving to older Latinos is expected to occur within the family. Among traditional Chicanos, an ethics of care calls for family members to guard the social and emotional well-being of parents and grandparents (Flores et al. 2009).

Aging is viewed as a normative process with concomitant decline and increasing dependence. The Latino ethics of care calls for elder autonomy, integrity, and independence to be honored and respected for as long as possible. Adult children are expected to find creative ways to preserve autonomy and dignity, while being called upon to assume increasing responsibility for the lives of their parents (see Flores et al. 2009).

Moreover, Chicano and Latino elders may expect their children and grandchildren to be involved in their lives, to afford them companionship and give them the status that their age, role in the family, and wisdom merit. However, due to migration, the acculturation of their children and grandchildren, and the changes in roles and developmental demands faced by US-born Latinos, adult children may not be as available for day-to-day companionship and support. Consequently, elders may feel cast aside and undervalued. The isolation of Latino older adults is a contributing factor to poor health, including depression and anxiety (Alford and Espino 2010). For older LGBTQ Latinos and Chicanos who lack family support, strong friendship networks and long-standing "families of choice" are essential to maintain and promote mental health (Espin 2012).

For men who socialized primarily through work, retirement or disability that leads to an interruption of their work life may contribute to lack of nonfamilial support systems. Losing the ability to drive, as is the case for those with cognitive decline, means loss of independence for many older adults. Increased dependence on family members, who may have limited time available to accompany them on errands or to simply be there, and social isolation are risk factors for depression and suicidality among older Chicanos (Hinton et al. 2009).

Given the structural and ecological realities faced by many older Chicanos, including a lifetime of low-paying, physically demanding, or dangerous work (farm work, construction, service sector jobs) with limited or no health insurance, many Chicanos reach the age when they should (or could) retire unable to do so. They may not have Social Security benefits or health insurance. Most Latino elders live below the poverty line and must continue to work or rely on family for subsistence. Such dependence may be a contributing factor to depression in older Chicano and Latino men.

As noted by Alford and Espino, important numbers of Mexican American women live alone, without the physical companionship of spouses or children. Without a traditional role to fulfill, many of these women can become depressed, especially if they experience the pain of arthritis or the disabling effects of hypertension or diabetes (Flores, Zelman, and Flores 2012).

A large number of older Chicanas are caregivers to parents, spouses, or in-laws affected by dementing illnesses, including Alzheimer's. Studies of Latina/o caregivers document that most Chicanas and Chicanos rely on familial rather than external sources of support (Apesoa-Varano, Barker, and Hinton 2011; Hinton et al. 2006; Flores et al. 2009). The experience of caregiving for parents or spouses with cognitive decline is stressful and associated with mood disorder, particularly if the elder is combative or aggressive or exhibits other behavioral symptoms of dementia (Hinton et al. 2006; Flores et al. 2009). Furthermore, most Latinos are not aware of the prevalence of dementing illnesses or that cognitive decline is associated with Alzheimer's disease and other degenerative dementias, not just with growing older. Likewise, many Latinos do not recognize the neuropsychiatric and behavioral symptoms of dementia and do not seek medication for their ill relative. Medication management may alleviate the symptoms and reduce patient suffering and caregiver stress (Apesoa-Varano et al. 2011; Hinton et al. 2006).

At a time when women may be able to enjoy a decreased responsibility in parenting, they may have to become parental figures to their parents, in-laws, or spouses. Balancing personal desires and obligations with the duty and desire to take care of aging and ill relatives may not be experienced as a burden, but it can be stressful (Flores et al. 2009). It can also increase economic stress, as family caregivers may need to forgo work to care for relatives. It is not uncommon to find older women with chronic illnesses (diabetes, hypertension) caring for aged, ill parents.

■ Vignette #17: "I didn't sign up for this"

Julieta is a fifty-nine-year-old, divorced, second-generation Chicana, who returned to California after living out of state for many years. Her older brother Juan asked her to return when their father began to show signs of cognitive decline. As Julieta did not have a husband and her children were grown, her brother felt she should return home to help their mother take care of their dad. Julieta sought therapy for herself, as she was becoming increasingly resentful of her caregiving duties. She had never gotten along with her dad, who was a traditional immigrant Mexican man who had disapproved of Julieta's life decisions. However, Julieta felt that it was her duty as a daughter to support her mother. Julieta's parents had immigrated to the United States when young; they had worked in agriculture all their lives and had never accessed adequate health care.

Juan had fought with multiple care providers until he was able to have his father diagnosed. When his father's primary care physician finally referred him to a specialist,[1] Juan decided to call Julieta. The brother and sister had agreed to split the caregiving duties. Juan paid for the care of his father, and Julieta moved in with them. However, after a few weeks, Julieta realized that she had "signed up" for more than she had imagined. Her father was combative, "uncooperative," and "macho." Julieta loved her mother and wanted to be of support but was becoming increasingly frustrated with her mother's dependence on her to control her husband. Julieta's mother had a heart condition and arthritis; she was frail and could not restrain her husband when he tried to leave the house. Julieta also worried that the stress of her father's illness was aggravating her own hypertension and diabetes. Just when Julieta had decided to focus on her health, she had to become her father's primary caregiver.

Julieta and her brother had researched Alzheimer's disease (AD) and understood that their father's behavioral problems and depression were associated with his illness. Yet Julieta expected her dad to have some control over his behavior. She attributed his combativeness and "willfulness" to *machismo*. Her father had been "old school" and authoritarian in his younger years. She saw his current behavior as an extension of his past conduct. She found herself yelling and screaming at him as she did when she was an adolescent. Subsequently, she felt guilty. She struggled with the obligation to be a good daughter and her desire to just run away, as she had when she married young and left home to escape her father's control. She saw it as ironic that once again, due to his illness, he had control over her life.

Unlike many Latinos and Chicanos who hold negative perceptions of mental health care and feel stigmatized when they seek such services,

Julieta felt she needed support, "a safe place to vent," where she could speak about her conflicted feelings about caring for her father, without fear of being judged as a bad daughter. Julieta was referred to a caregiver support group; she also invited her brother to a few sessions of family therapy so that she could ask directly for more involvement from him and his wife and children in the day-to-day care of their father. Building a closer connection among family members also allowed for them to share their grief about losing their father to AD and to voice their fears and concerns about their caregiving responsibilities.

■ Depression among Elderly Chicana/os

It is estimated that about 5 percent of adults aged fifty-five or older in the United States will experience mild to moderate depression (Choi and Kim 2007). As stated in earlier chapters, Latinas have higher rates of depression than Latinos and white non-Hispanic women. However, in recent studies of aging, high rates of undiagnosed and untreated depression were found among Mexican-origin and Chicano men (Hinton, Chambers, and Velasquez 2009).

Depression late in life has been associated with morbidity and mortality (Alford and Espino 2010). The Sacramento Area Study on Aging (SALSA) (Gonzalez, Haan, and Hinton 2001; Haan et al. 2003) established the overall rate of depression for Latinos at 25.4 percent for US-born Mexican Americans in the sample; immigrant Latinos had a higher rate of 30.4 percent. The depression rates for women were significantly higher, 32 percent, compared to 16.3 percent for the men in the SALSA study. Greater risk for depression was found among the least-acculturated men and women (Gonzalez, Haan, and Hinton 2001).

More recently Hinton et al. (2009) found that when an older Latino male was depressed, his cognitive functioning was affected and that his spouse was more likely to become depressed as well. However, spousal depression did not affect Latino males. This finding may reflect the influence of gender roles on caregiving and the impact of family distress on Chicanas' emotional well-being.

As with other mental health problems, the patient's explanatory model will influence how an older Latino/a understands his or her symptoms and whether or not professional care is sought. The symptoms of depression may not be understood by the men as biomedical in nature; instead, they may use metaphors of loss and disappointment to describe their mood. Mr. Lopez and don Sebastian (chapter 4) held traditional roles and saw their worth as men anchored in providing for their families. When they were unable to work due to illness or disability, they experienced a loss of agency and self-valuation. Likewise, growing older and facing physical limitations as a result of arthritis or diabetes can challenge men's self-perceptions. Unless men can find alternative ways to contribute to the family and find meaning in the experience of aging, mood and anxiety disorders may occur. If the family cannot reframe the losses as normative to aging *or* provide a useful role to the Latino elder, he may feel helpless and become hopeless, which in turn can affect his physical, emotional, and spiritual health.

Likewise the idioms of distress utilized by older and less acculturated Latinos may result in physician lack of understanding of the patients' reports or accounts of his illness. For instance, Hinton et al. (2009) found that physicians were less likely to diagnose older Latinos as depressed, perhaps due to the patients' descriptions of their distress. Often the men indicated they felt useless rather than describing a sad mood.

■ Understanding Dementia

As stated earlier, the prevalence of dementing illnesses among Latinos is equal to or higher than among white non-Hispanics (Alford and Espino 2010; Applewhite, Garcia Biggs, and Herrera 2010). According to the *DSM-IV-TR,* dementia is a clinical syndrome characterized by cognitive impairment, which represents a decline from a higher level of functioning (Hinton et al. 2009). Cognitive impairment entails short-term memory loss and diminished executive functioning (performing tasks that include planning and sequencing; the ability to make decisions and exercise judgment), as well as difficulties with expressive and receptive language (aphasia— impairment in the expression and understanding of language, diminished capacity to read and write; apraxia—the inability to perform movement or use the correct words as a result of brain injury or disorder; or agnosia— the inability to recognize faces, people, or places).

Degenerative dementias, which are a subtype of dementia, include vascular dementia and Alzheimer's disease. In addition to cognitive impairment, there are important behavioral changes and neuropsychiatric symptoms that are of concern (although these are not part of the diagnostic criteria of the *DSM-IV-TR*). Most studies of family caregivers find that it is the disruptive behavioral changes—increased agitation, combativeness, willfulness, and the psychiatric symptoms (hallucinations, delusions, paranoia)—which are most distressing to family members and caregivers (Apesoa-Varano, Barker, and Hinton 2011; Hinton et al. 2009).

Latinos tend to utilize an explanatory model that relies on both biomedical and cultural explanations to account for the neuropsychiatric changes that accompany AD or other forms of dementia in their loved ones. In their study of older Latinos, Gallagher-Thompson and colleagues (1997) found that Latinos often stigmatize older Latinos in the early stages of dementia and label their behavior as "crazy." Other researchers find that Latinos consider cognitive decline, especially memory loss, as a sign of normal aging. However, they struggle with the behavioral and psychiatric symptoms of degenerative dementias (Novak and Riggs 2004). Even when they have access to information regarding dementia, family members may still attribute behavioral changes to character or personality or consider the "troublesome behaviors" to be under the ill relative's control (see Apesoa-Varano, Barker, and Hinton 2011; Hinton et al. 2006).

However, family responses to the symptoms of AD may not reflect the explanatory model of the caregiver or family. For example, in an ethnographic study of six Mexican American caregivers of husbands with dementia, Apesoa-Varano, Barker, and Hinton (2011) found that all spousal caregivers relied on family members, typically their sons or daughters, to help manage the behavioral problems of their husbands. Furthermore, even when they understood that their relative's problematic behavior was a symptom of the illness, they responded to the behavior as if it were in the care recipient's control, as did Julia, who believed her father could control his belligerent and combative behavior. In one of the case studies from the sample, the wife threatened her husband with calling her sons to "punish" him for his misbehavior. While the family understood that the aggressive behavior was a symptom of AD, they acted as if he had some control over his behavior, and they became frustrated by his symptoms.

At times, caregivers who have lower levels of acculturation may attribute the neuropsychiatric symptoms or behavioral problems to traits or character. Hinton et al. (2006) and Flores et al. (2009) studies of Latino caregivers of elders with dementia found that immigrant spouses, and daughters with low acculturation, tended to attribute the behavioral problems of the care recipient as rooted in personality traits: "she was always selfish and willful; now she is just more so"; "she was always a stressed-out person, and now she is just more anxious"; "he always had an ill temper (*ser corajudo*), and now he doesn't try to hold back." Other family members attributed the cognitive decline and the depression associated with AD to having lived a hard life. The suffering endured had finally caught up with the elder.

Others may attribute the behavioral and psychiatric symptoms as a result of susto, which can be triggered by interpersonal stress or receiving bad news (Applewhite, Garcia Biggs, and Herrera 2010). The Soto family associated their mother's early symptoms of AD with the news that her own mother had died in Mexico. Mrs. Soto migrated to the United States as a young woman. She did not obtain legal status in the United States until her children were grown; thus, she was not able to see her mother for over thirty years. When she was preparing for her first trip to Mexico to see her mother, Mrs. Soto received news that her mother had suffered a stroke and died. Mrs. Soto "*se puso fuera de si.*" According to her children, Mrs. Soto lost touch with reality. While they acknowledged that she had become increasingly forgetful and that they had observed subtle personality changes over the previous two years, it was the bad news that led to her "locura." Mrs. Soto's children and husband were embarrassed by her behavior and did not tell her physician about it when she had regular visits to manage her hypertension and diabetes. They wanted to protect her from the opinions of others (el que dirán). It was not until she began to wander about the neighborhood and get lost, and when she ceased speaking, that they told the doctor about their concerns. It was then that Mrs. Soto was diagnosed with AD.

While more-acculturated children struggle with balancing the love and obligation to their parents and their own individual desires, immigrant Latina daughters and daughters-in-law as well as spousal caregivers tended to demonstrate selfless devotion to their ill parent or spouse. They held on to traditional views of filial devotion and marital commitment (see Flores et al. 2009).

■ Vignette #18: "*Su historia es mi historia*" (Her story is my story)

Mr. Ruiz was a sixty-year-old Mexican man who had immigrated to the United States at age nineteen. He lived in rural northern California. He had made the United States his home and had visited Mexico only twice: the first time to find a wife in the rural village where he was born, and the second to seek a curandera to help his wife when she began to show signs of what was later diagnosed as AD.

Mr. Ruiz was interviewed as part of a qualitative study of Latina/o caregivers of relatives with dementia (Hinton et al. 2006). He told us about his life when he first came to California. As he faced extreme racism, he decided never to have children. He wanted to spare a new generation what he had faced—poverty and lack of opportunity in Mexico and racism in the United States. When he was about thirty, he went to Mexico to find a wife. He met a young woman in his rancho who agreed to marry him and not to have children. The two settled in a rural Northern California community, where he worked and she was a housewife. She was a gifted seamstress and made clothes for other Mexican and Chicano families in their town. Mr. Ruiz described his marriage as solid; they created a home filled with love and the smells of her cooking and the beauty of her sewing. He never wanted to visit Mexico, so he often sent for her mother and sisters to visit.

When his wife was in her late forties, she began to show signs of depression. She did not want to go out to visit friends, and he found her asleep sometimes when he arrived home from work. Typically, she would have dinner ready for him. At first he thought she was tired, but later he began to think that she was "going through the change." He read a lot and knew that sometimes women become depressed during menopause. When he asked her about her mood, she denied feeling sad. When Mrs. Ruiz was in her early fifties, Mr. Ruiz came home and found her asleep with the stove on. He awoke her and she seemed not to know where she was. One day he discovered that she had hidden a lot of cloth that she was supposed to convert into dresses for a quinceañera. When he asked her about it, she seemed confused.

Mr. Ruiz took his wife to the doctor, who concurred that she was probably depressed. Over the next few months, some of the neighbors began to call him at work with concerns about his wife's behavior. Previously a sweet and kind lady, she was at times rude and would refuse to open the door for them when they came to visit. Mr. Ruiz invited one of his sisters-in-law from Mexico to come stay with his wife, thinking that this would improve his wife's mood. However, his sister-in-law became very alarmed at Mrs. Ruiz's condition. She was refusing to bathe or change clothes. The family in Mexico began to question Mr. Ruiz and accused him of mistreating his wife. He became upset and sent his sister-in-law back to Mexico.

Mr. Ruiz took early retirement to stay with his wife and monitor her behavior. At his mother-in-law's urging, he took his wife to Mexico to see a curandera. However, his wife's condition did not improve. Her cognitive abilities continued to decline, and her behavior became more erratic. Mr. Ruiz became very upset that he had agreed to take his wife to a curandera, as he did not believe it would help. His wife's family perceived as maltreatment his unwillingness to leave her in Mexico to continue receiving treatment from healers there. He brought his wife back to the United States and broke all communication with her family.

Upon the couple's return from Mexico, Mr. Ruiz insisted that his wife be reevaluated. She was referred to a specialist, who diagnosed her with AD. Mr. Ruiz was devastated. He took care of his wife at home for two years but, finding it increasingly difficult to manage her at home, he then placed her in a convalescent home. His wife stopped speaking. At the time of the interview with our research team, Mrs. Ruiz had been in the facility for nearly a year. Mr. Ruiz visited her every day; he fed her breakfast and then returned home to "putter around." He returned to the facility to feed her lunch and, later, dinner. He stayed with his wife every evening until she fell asleep.

Mr. Ruiz was a traditional man who appeared stoic. He denied any depression or anxiety. He worried about his wife and felt guilty about having her in the facility; he believed that she was angry at him for putting her there and that this was why she did not speak. He was in relatively good health and expressed a desire to take a vacation, but did not want to leave his wife.

He had become increasingly isolated as the neighbors and former friends had been critical of his wife's locura and encouraged him to rebuild his life. He was outraged. As he put it, "Her story is my story. She can no longer enjoy our life, so I will be with her until the good Lord takes her." Having no children who could step in and help out, he saw caring for his wife as his duty. "I married her for better or for worse," he said. "This is the 'for worse' part."

We found few male spousal caregivers in our study. Mr. Ruiz was unique in that he had no family to help him with caregiving; he had refused his sister-in-law's offer of help and the request that his wife be sent to Mexico. He wanted her to have access to good health care. That was a factor in his decision to keep her in the United States and place her in a facility. However, his behavior reflected his cultural values of loyalty and obligation.

Summary

As stated, Latino cultural norms call for families to attend to the psychosocial needs of their aging relatives. To the extent that family members retain these values across generations and levels of acculturation, caregiving will continue to occur in the home whenever possible, with relatives as providers of care. Given the low income and limited health care access characteristic of many Latinos and Chicanos, families will need support to carry out their ethics of care when their own health is compromised.

Prevention of chronic illness and access to adequate care when illnesses first appear would do much to improve the health and quality of life of Chicanos as they age. Educational campaigns about comorbid conditions and their impact on the emotional and spiritual health of caregivers and care recipients are needed. Above all, a better understanding of the experience of aging among Chicanos is required to develop appropriate interventions to increase well-being en la tercera edad.

Discussion Questions

1. What are the leading causes of death for older Latinos?

2. How do Chicanos typically explain the behavioral problems of elderly persons with dementia?

3. What is the association between diabetes, depression, and cognitive decline?

4. How may familial caregivers be supported in their caregiving role?

Note

1. See Hinton et al. (2006) for an account of the multiple barriers Latino families face in trying to obtain appropriate diagnosis and treatment of parents with degenerative dementias.

Suggested Readings

Applewhite, Steven R., Mary Jo Garcia Biggs, and Angelica P. Herrera. "Health and Mental Health Perspectives on Elderly Latinos in the United States." In *Health Issues in Latino Males, ed.* Marilyn Aguirre-Molina, Luisa N. Borrell, and William Vega, 235–49. New Brunswick, NJ: Rutgers University Press, 2010.

Flores, Yvette. "Embodying Dementia: Remembrances of Memory Loss." In *Speaking from the Body: Latinas on Health and Culture*. ed. Angie Chabram-Dernersesian and Adela de la Torre, 31–43. Tucson: University of Arizona Press, 2008.

Flores, Yvette G., Ladson Hinton, Judith C. Barker, Carol E. Franz, Alexandra Velasquez. "Beyond Familism: Ethics of Care of Latina Caregivers of Elderly Parents with Dementia." *Health Care for Women International* 30, no. 12 (2009): 1055–72.

González, Hector M., Mary Haan, and Ladson Hinton. "Acculturation and the Prevalence of Depression in Older Mexican Americans: Baseline Results of the Sacramento Area Latino Study on Aging." *Journal of the American Geriatric Society* 49, no. 7 (2001): 948–53.

Haan, Mary M., Dan M. Mungas, Hector M. Gonzalez, Teresa A. Ortiz, Ananth Acharya, and William J. Jagust. "Prevalence of Dementia in Older Latinos: The Influence of Type 2 Diabetes Mellitus, Stroke and Genetic Factors." *Journal of the American Geriatric Society* 51, no. 2 (2003): 169–77.

Hinton, Ladson, Darren Chambers, and Alexandra Velasquez. "Making Sense of Behavioral Disturbances in Persons with Dementia: Latino Family Caregiver Attributions of Neuropsychiatric Inventory Domains." *Alzheimer Disease and Associated Disorders* 23, no. 4 2009: 401–5.

Hinton, Ladson, Yvette Flores, Carol Franz, Isabel Hernandez, and Linda S. Mitteness. "The Borderlands of Primary Care: Physician and Family Perspectives on 'Troublesome Behaviors' of People with Dementia." In *Thinking about Dementia: Culture, Loss, and the Anthropology of Senility,* ed. Annette Leibing and Lawrence Cohen, 43–63. New Brunswick, NJ: Rutgers University Press, 2006.

Hinton, Ladson, Yolanda Hagar, Nancy West, Hector M. González, Dan Mungas, Laurel Beckett, and Mary N. Haan. "Longitudinal Influence of Partner Depression on Cognitive Functioning in Latino Spousal Pairs." *Dementia and Geriatric Cognitive Disorders* 27, no. 6 (2009): 491–500.

Conclusion

Chicana/o Mental Health in the Twenty-First Century

The growth of the Chicano population over the past two decades and the entry of Latino professionals into positions of authority in the fields of health, mental health, education, and policy have increased the interest in understanding and promoting the well-being of Mexican-origin people. The chapters in this book offer a comprehensive view of the mental health needs of US-born *mexicanas y mexicanos*. Utilizing a life-cycle perspective, the mental health problems of children, adolescents, adults, and seniors are examined, foregrounding the importance of taking into account the cultural explanatory models utilized by Chicanas and Chicanos as well as more biomedical views of the causes of problemas del alma, la mente, y el corazón.

By most accounts, most Chicanas and Chicanos experience economic, social, educational, and health disparities that are largely the result of decades of inequality (Carlo et al. 2009; Vega, Borrell, and Aguirre-Molina 2010). Such disparities increase the risk for academic disengagement in children, and family stress that can lead to child-rearing problems, which in turn adds to the acculturative stress of adolescents and young adults. When the American Dream does not materialize, generation after generation, Chicano men become susceptible to substance misuse, violence, and despair. Women and children often receive the sequelae of such despair through neglect, maltreatment, abandonment, and violence. Both men and women struggle at times with competing cultural mandates and expectations. The mental health problems of adult Chicanos and Chicanas are multidetermined. However, increased attention to social inequalities and their multigenerational effects is essential to improve the emotional well-being of Chicanos (Portes, Fernandez-Kelly, and Haller 2005; Rumbaut 1994).

Promoting Balance *en el Alma, la Mente, y el Corazón*

The studies reviewed in this book offer strategies for addressing the risk factors faced by Chicana and Chicano children and youth. Cultural protective factors—family cohesion, a balance of cargas y regalos, age-appropriate responsibilities as children grow, and *rooting* the children in the positive aspects of their culture of origin can do much to build pride in their ethnicity and thereby buffer the inevitable racial, ethnic, and gender microaggressions Chicanos will experience outside the home. Supporting families in their efforts to raise children who will follow the good path and thus enjoy the good life is equally important. Parents need support in order to raise bicultural children healthy in body, mind, and spirit.

Countering and reducing the increased risk for depression, anxiety, substance misuse, and violence in adolescence and adulthood necessitate educational changes and increased access to prevention and promotion programs that are culturally attuned and respond to the diversity of Chicanos. The research findings reviewed in this book document the emotional and psychological toll caused by societal pressures to acculturate, lack of family support for biculturality, and increased xenophobia and intolerance. Often the larger society and the family mirror Chicano youth disparagement, disapproval, despair. Community-based programs rooted in Chicano cultures and traditions aim to mirror positive reflections of pride in ancestral culture and thereby find cultural solutions to imbalance.

As Chicanas and Chicanos mature and find their own paths, the cargas y regalos given by the family can guide or impede their progress and well-being. As the vignettes presented in this book indicate, acculturated, educated Chicanos also are at risk for depression, anxiety, and substance misuse. Society mirrors back to them as well that no matter what they attain, what positions they hold, they are at risk for stereotyping, discrimination, and psychological assault. To maintain well-being the spirit must be strengthened through awareness, *concientización* (raising consciousness), that racism harms and that microaggressions deplete emotional energy and can lead to rage and despair. As the indigenous ancestors taught, finding meaning in experience and understanding one's destino are crucial for emotional and physical health (Duran and Duran 1995; Ramirez 1998). Families and schools can do much to guide the child and youth to find his and her destino and can inoculate Chicanos against the multiple forms of marginalization and discrimination to which they will be exposed in their lifetimes.

Chicanas and Chicanos of all generations are influenced by cultural values; cultural scripts can be sources of support—familism, or reliance on family, which can provide social and emotional support—or sources of distress—fulfilling cultural mandates without having the economic or emotional resources to do so, for example, caregiving of frail elderly while having to work and raise a family (Flores et al. 2009). Moreover, understanding cultural values and how they visibly and invisibly impact behavior can be a powerful healing tool.

While this book does not offer recommendations for treatment, I do argue that to engage Chicanos in therapy requires a careful assessment of their generational level, cultural adherence, ethnic identity, language preference, explanatory model of health and illness, and exposure to microaggressions, as well as their history of violence (Bernal and Flores-Ortiz 1982; Bernal, Flores-Ortiz, and Rodriguez-Dragin 1986). Such an assessment, along with the mental health provider's cultural attunement, can facilitate joining and increase the likelihood that the client will remain in treatment long enough to explore the roots of his or her distress and develop adaptive ways of healing the body, mind, and heart.

■ Policy Implications of Latina/o Mental Health Status

A number of community organizations have created programs over the past four decades that address directly the mental health needs of Chicanos of various generations. These programs have been successful; they counter underutilization with outreach, community education, and programs that respond to community needs with respect to culture, language, ancestry, and diversity. These organizations also provide training to students, young professionals, and *promotores* in order to serve their clients utilizing both western psychological and indigenous tools (see Clinica de la Raza and Instituto Familiar de la Raza as examples in Northern California). These agencies often are underfunded and struggle to remain viable. To address the needs of the growing Latino population requires adequate funding and a commitment to improve the lives of all Chicanos.

The research findings reviewed in this book underscore the importance of improving the mental health of Chicanos of all ages. Social isolation and poor physical health in the last third of life are reflective of the challenges Chicanos faced in their lifetimes—health disparities, and low income resulting from undereducation and limited employment opportunities. Yet Chicano elders emerge as resilient and hopeful, despite the difficulties they experienced in life. While they report that their health is poor, they find meaning in their role as elders; when family support is absent, that meaning is less protective (Applewhite, Garcia Biggs, and Herrera 2010; Hinton et al. 2009).

Clearly, within the Chicano cultural value system, each stage of life requires having a place—psychological rootedness—and finding meaning. Families and communities must work together with government support to create safety and meaningful opportunities for Chicanos. As the US population ages, Chicanos will constitute the workforce that contributes to those elders' economic and social well-being. An important question is raised: Who will take care of Chicana/os when they are elders? When today's Chicano twenty-year-olds enter their third stage of life, they will constitute the majority of people over sixty. Will a social security system exist to reward them for decades of work? What are the implications of increased incarceration for Chicano youth? Chicanos can build a solid foundation for the future of this country; however, such a foundation must be built on well-funded schools and strategies that promote good mental, physical, and spiritual health. Researchers have illuminated the path to increased well-being for Latinos in this country. It is up to policy makers and well-informed Latinos to ensure that the light continues to shine, guiding future generations of Chicanos toward balance in alma, mente, y corazón.

■ Toward Cultural Humility and Professional Training

Health professionals play a key role in promoting and maintaining well-being. Cultural respect, humility, and attunement are essential elements in engagement, evaluation, and treatment of Latino clients or patients (de La Torre and Estrada 2001). The American Psychological Association responded to the demands of psychologists of color to include respect for diversity in race, gender, and culture as ethical responsibilities for the profession. Consequently, training programs have responded with increased training opportunities and enhanced curriculum. When I was a graduate student in the 1970s, a course on "multicultural psychology" might be offered now and again. I had to seek training outside my graduate institution to gain experience providing services to Latinos and African Americans. Today, more courses are available. However, much remains to be done. Marginalization of professionals of color continues, not enough Latinos enter "the helping and healing" professions (as indicated in the introduction to this book). Insufficient numbers of non-Latino professionals gain adequate training to work with diverse Latino groups. An educated Latino workforce is essential; likewise increased numbers of mental health practitioners who are culturally and linguistically attuned to diverse Chicano/Latino groups are needed to address Chicana/o mental health needs (see Bernal and Domenech Rodriguez 2012).

This book offers a model of understanding Chicano mental health needs that is respectful of Chicano diversity; while rooted in the importance of knowing and connecting to the past, it recognizes the need to critically examine existing treatment models and develop Chicano and Latino best practices (see Bernal, Sáez-Santiago, and Galloza-Carrero 2009; Muñoz et al. 2010; Organista 2007; Szapocznik et al. 1989). The mental health needs of Chicanas and Chicanos are many. Their cultural capital—resilience in the face of adversity and historical trauma—also must be acknowledged and better understood.

In the 1970s Chicano professionals concluded that *la cultura cura* (culture heals); this was a call to root oneself again in the healing ways of our indigenous ancestors—to identify cultural values and traditions that had healing potential and to teach those to the next generation. Finding meaning in one's destiny, identifying ways to promote and maintain balance and to be accountable to the next seven generations, can promote health and maximize the human potential of this nation's largest ethnic group. *Con respeto* (with respect), I offer this book.

■ WORKS CITED

Aguilar-Gaxiola, Sergio A., Lynnette Zelezny, Betty Garcia, Christine Edmonson, Christina Alejo-Garcia, and William A. Vega. "Translating Research into Action: Reducing Disparities in Mental Health Care for Mexican Americans." *Psychiatric Services* 53, no. 12 (2002): 1563–68.

Aguirre-Molina, Marilyn, and Gabriela Betancourt. "Latino Boys: The Early Years." In Aguirre-Molina, Borrell, and Vega, *Health Issues in Latino Males,* 67–82.

Aguirre-Molina, Marilyn, Luisa N. Borrell, Miguel Muñoz-Laboy, and William Vega. "Introduction: A Social and Structural Framework for the Analysis of Latino Males' Health." In Aguirre-Molina, Borrell, and Vega, *Health Issues in Latino Males,* 1–16.

Aguirre-Molina, Marilyn, Luisa N. Borrell, and William Vega, eds. *Health Issues in Latino Males.* New Brunswick, NJ: Rutgers University Press, 2010.

Alderete, Ethel, William A. Vega, Bohdan Kolody, and Sergio A. Aguilar-Gaxiola. "Lifetime Prevalence of and Risk Factors for Psychiatric Disorders among Mexican Migrant Farmworkers in California." *American Journal of Public Health* 90, no. 4 (2000): 608–14.

Alegria, Margarita, M. Atkins, E. Farmer, E. Slaton, and W. Stelk. "One Size Does Not Fit All: Taking Diversity, Culture and Context Seriously." *Administration and Policy in Mental Health and Mental Health Services Research* 37, nos. 1–2 (2010): 48–60.

Alegria, Margarita, Glorisa Canino, Patrick E. Shrout, Meghan Woo, Nahiua Duan, Doryliz Vila, Maria Torres, Chih-Nan Chen, and Xiao-Li Meng. "Prevalence of Mental Illness in Immigrant and Non-Immigrant U.S. Latino Groups." *American Journal of Psychiatry* 165, no. 3 (2008): 359–69.

Alegria, Margarita, Norah Mulvaney-Day, Maria Torres, Antonio Polo, Zhun Cao, and Glorisa Canino. "Prevalence of Psychiatric Disorders across Latino Subgroups in the United States." *American Journal of Public Health* 97, no. 1 (2007): 68–75.

Alegria, Margarita, William Scribney, Meghan Woo, Maria Torres, and Peter Guarnaccia. "Looking beyond Nativity: The Relation of Age of Immigration, Length of Residence, and Birth Cohorts to the Risk of Onset of Psychiatric Disorders for Latinos." *Journal of Research in Human Development* 4, no. 1 (2007): 19–47.

Alegria, Margarita, David Takeuchi, Glorisa Canino, Naihua Duan, Patrick E. Shrout, Xiao-Li Meng, Nolan Zane, Doryliz Vila, Meghan Woo, Mildred Vera, Peter Guarnaccia, Sergio Aguilar-Gaxiola, Stanley Sue, Javier Escobar, Keh-ming Lin, and Fong Gong. "Considering Context, Place and Culture: The National Latino and Asian American Study." *International Journal of Methods in Psychiatric Research* 13, no. 4 (2004): 208–20.

Alegria, Margarita, and Meghan Woo. "Conceptual Issues in Latino Mental Health." In Villaruel et al., *Handbook of U.S. Latino Psychology: Developmental and Community-Based Perspectives,* 15–30.

Alford, Cynthia, and David Espino. "Mental Health of Elderly Latino Males." In Aguirre-Molina, Borrell, and Vega, *Health Issues in Latino Males,* 249–60.

Almaguer, Tomas. "Chicano Men: A Cartography of Homosexual Identity and Behavior." In *The Lesbian and Gay Studies Reader,* edited by Henry Abelove and Michèle Aina Barale, 255–73. New York: Routledge, 1993.

Almeida, Rhea. *Transformations of Gender and Race: Family and Developmental Perspectives.* New York: Haworth, 1998.

———. "What Straight Therapists Can Do." *Family Magazine* 2, no. 4 (1997): 7–11.

Almeida, Rhea, Ken Dolan-Del Vecchio, and Lynn Parker. "Foundation Concepts for Social Justice Based Therapy: Critical Consciousness, Accountability, and Empowerment." In *Promoting Social Justice through Mental Health Practice,* ed. Etiony Aldarondo, 175–206. Mahwah, NJ: Lawrence Erlbaum, 2007.

Almeida, Rhea, and Judith Lockard. "The Cultural Context Model: A New Paradigm for Accountability, Empowerment and the Development of Critical Consciousness against Domestic Violence." In *Domestic Violence at the Margins: Readings on Race, Class, Gender and Culture,* ed. Natalie J. Sokoloff and Christina Pratt, 301–20. New Brunswick, NJ: Rutgers University Press, 2005.

Almeida, Rhea, Theresa Messineo, Rosemary Woods, and Robert Font. "Violence in the Lives of the Racially and Sexually Different: A Public and Private Dilemma." In *Expansions of Feminist Family Therapy through Diversity,* ed. Rhea Almeida, 99–134. London: Psychology Press, 1994.

American Psychiatric Association. *Diagnostic and Statistical Manual of Mental Disorders (DSM-IV-TR),* 4th ed. Washington, DC: American Psychiatric Association, 2000.

American Psychological Association. "Principles of Psychologists and Code of Conduct." Washington, DC: American Psychological Association, 2010.

Anzaldúa, Gloria. *Borderlands/La Frontera: The New Mestiza.* San Francisco: Spinsters/Aunt Lute, 1987.

Apesoa-Varano, Ester C., Judith C. Barker, Carol Franz, and Ladson Hinton. "Curing and Caring: The Work of Primary Care Physicians with Dementia Patients." *Qualitative Health Research,* September 26, 2011. http://qhr.sagepub.com/content/early/2011/06/16/1049732311412788.

Apesoa-Varano, C., Judith C. Barker, and Ladson Hinton. "Mexican-American Families and Dementia: An Exploration of "Work" in Response to Dementia-Related Aggressive Behavior." In *Aging, Health and Longevity in the Mexican-Origin Population,* ed. Jacqueline L. Angel, Fernando Torres-Gil, and Kyriakos Markides, 277–92. New York: Springer, 2011.

Applewhite, Steven R., Mary Jo Garcia Biggs, and Angelica P. Herrera. "Health and Mental Health Perspectives on Elderly Latinos in the United States." In Aguirre-Molina, Borrell, and Vega, *Health Issues in Latino Males,* 235–49.

Arellano, Leticia H. "A Subculture of a Culture: A Hermeneutic Study of the Latina/o-Chicana/o Punk Experience." PhD diss., Wright Institute Graduate School of Psychology, Berkeley, 2011.

Arévalo, Sandra P., Laia Bécares, and Hortencia Amaro. "The Health of Incarcerated Latino Men." In Aguirre-Molina, Borrell, and Vega, *Health Issues in Latino Males,* 139–57.

Avila, Elena, and Joy Parker. *Woman Who Glows in the Dark: A Curandera Reveals Traditional Aztec Secrets of Physical and Spiritual Health.* New York: J. P. Tarcher/Putnam, 2000.

Ayala, George. "Balancing Research with Rights-Based Principles of Practice for Programming for Men Who Have Sex with Men." *Spotlight on Prevention,* May 3, 2012, *USAID.* http://www.aidstar-one.com/focus_areas/prevention/resources/spotlight/balancing_research_rights_based_principles_practice_programming_men_who_have_sex_men.

———. "Social Determinants of HIV/AIDS: A Focus on Discrimination and Latino Men Who Have Sex with Men." In Aguirre-Molina, Borrell, and Vega, *Health Issues in Latino Males,* 212–28.

Ayala, George, and Rafael M. Diaz. "Racism, Poverty and Other Truths about Sex: Race, Class and HIV Risk among Latino Gay Men." *Revista Interamericana de Psicologia* 35, no. 2 (2001): 59–77.

Ayala, Jennifer. "Confianza, Consejos and Contradictions: Gender and Sexuality Lessons between Latina Adolescent Daughters and Mothers." In *Latina Girls: Voices of Strength in the United States,* ed. Jill Denner and Bianca L. Guzmán, 29–43. New York: New York University Press, 2006.

Azmitia, Margarita, and Jane R. Brown. "Latino Immigrant Parents' Beliefs about 'The Path of Life' of Their Adolescent Children." In *Latino Children and Families in the United States: Current Research and Future Directions,* ed. Josefina M. Contreras, Kathryn A. Kearns, and Angela M. Neal-Barnett, 77–106. Westport, CT: Praeger, 2002.

Baker Miller, Jean. *Towards a New Psychology of Women.* Boston: Beacon Press, 1974.

Baptiste, David A. Jr., Kenneth V. Hardy, and Laurie Lewis. "Family Therapy with English Caribbean Immigrant Families in the United States: Issues of Emigration, Immigration, Culture, and Race." *Contemporary Family Therapy* 19, no. 3 (1997): 337–59.

Barrera, Manuel Jr., Nancy A. Gonzales, Vera Lopez, and A. Cristina Fernandez. "Problem Behaviors of Chicana/o and Latina/o Adolescents: An Analysis of Prevalence, Risk, and Protective Factors." In *The Handbook of Chicana/o Psychology and Mental Health,* ed. Roberto Velazquez, Leticia Arellano, and Brian McNeill, 83–110. Mahwah, NJ: Lawrence Erlbaum, 2004.

Barrera, Manuel Jr., Devon N. Hageman, and Nancy A. Gonzales. "Revisiting Hispanic Adolescents' Resilience to the Effects of Parental Problem Drinking and Life Stress." *American Journal of Community Psychology* 34, nos. 1–2 (2004): 1–2.

Bauer, Heidi, Michael A. Rodriguez, Seline Szkupinski Quiroga, and Yvette G. Flores-Ortiz. "Barriers to Health Care for Abused Latinas and Asian Immigrant Women." *Journal of Health Care for the Poor and the Underserved* 11, no. 1 (2000): 33–44.

Bernal, Guillermo, and Melanie M. Domenech Rodriguez, eds. *Cultural Adaptations: Tools for Evidence-Based Practice with Diverse Populations.* Washington, DC: American Psychological Association, 2012.

Bernal, Guillermo, and Yvette Flores-Ortiz. "Contextual Family Therapy with Adolescent Drug Abusers." In *Family Therapy Approaches with Adolescent Substance Abusers,* ed. Thomas C. Todd, 70–92. New York: Allyn and Bacon, 1990.

———. "Latino Families in Therapy: Engagement and Evaluation." *Journal of Marital and Family Therapy* 8, no. 3 (1982): 357–65.

Bernal, Guillermo, Yvette Flores-Ortiz, and Carmenza Rodriguez-Dragin. "Terapia familiar intergeneracional con chicanos y familias mejicanas inmigrantes a los Estados Unidos" (Contextual family therapy with Chicanos and Mexican immigrants). *Cuadernos de Psicología* 8, no. 1 (1986): 81–99.

Bernal, Guillermo, Emily Saez-Santiago, and Amarilys Galloza-Carrero. "Evidence-Based Approaches to Working with Latino Youth and Families." In Villaruel et al., *Handbook of U.S. Latino Psychology: Developmental and Community-Based Perspectives,* 309–28.

Bernal, Marta E., and George P. Knight, eds. *Ethnic Identity: Formation and Transmission among Hispanics and Other Minorities.* Albany: State University of New York Press, 1993.

Beyene, Yewoubdar, Gay Becker, and Nury Mayen. "Perception of Aging and Sense of Well-Being among Latino Elderly." *Journal of Cross-Cultural Gerontology* 17, no. 2 (2002): 155–72.

Biggs, M. Antonia, Claire D. Brindis, Lauren Ralph, and John Santelli. "The Sexual and Reproductive Health of Young Latino Males Living in the United States." In Aguirre-Molina, Borrell, and Vega, *Health Issues in Latino Males,* 83–98.

Bird, Hector R., Glorisa Canino, Maritza Rubio-Stipek, Madelyn S. Gould, Julio C. Ribera, and Myrna Sesman. "Estimates of the Prevalence of Childhood Maladjustment in a Community Survey in Puerto Rico." *Archives of General Psychiatry* 45, no. 9 (1988): 1120–26.

Bird, Hector R., Thomas J. Yager, Beatriz Staghezza, Madelyn S. Gould, Glorisa Canino, and Maritza Rubio-Stipec. "Impairment in the Epidemiological Measurement of Childhood Psychopathology in the Community." *Journal of the American Academy of Child and Adolescent Psychiatry* 28, no. 6 (1990): 847–50.

Breitborde, Nicholas J., Steven R. Lopez, and Alex Kopelowicz. "Expressed Emotion and Health Outcomes among Mexican Americans with Schizophrenia and Their Caregivers." *Journal of Nervous and Mental Disease* 198, no. 2 (2010): 105–9.

Burnette, Denise. "Custodial Grandparents in Latino Families: Patterns of Service Use and Predictors of Unmet Needs." *Social Work* 44, no. 1 (1999): 22–34.

Caetano, Raul, Jonali Baruah, Suhasini Ramisetty-Mikler, and Malembe S. Ebama. "Sociodemographic Predictors of Pattern and Volume of Alcohol Consumption across Hispanics, Blacks, and Whites: 10-Year Trend (1992–2002)." *Alcoholism: Clinical and Experimental Research* 34, no. 10 (2010): 1782–92.

Caetano, Raul, Craig Field, Suhasini Ramisetty, and Sherry Lipsky. "Agreement on Reporting of Physical, Psychological, and Sexual Violence among White, Black, and Hispanic Couples in the United States." *Journal of Interpersonal Violence* 24, no. 8 (2009): 1318–37.

Caldera, Yvonne M., Jacki Fitzpatrick, and Karen S. Wampler. "Coparenting in Intact Mexican American Families: Mothers' and Fathers' Perceptions." In *Latino Children and Families in the United States: Current Research and Future Directions,* ed. Josefina M. Contreras, Kathryn A. Kearns, and Angela M. Neal-Barnett, 107–32. Westport, CT: Praeger, 2002.

Caldwell, Amelia, Amy Couture, and Heidi Nowotny. *Closing the Mental Health Gap: Eliminating Disparities in Treatment for Latinos.* Kansas City: Mattie Rhodes Center, 2008.

Candelaria, Cordelia. "La Malinche: Feminist Prototype." *Frontiers: A Journal of Women Studies* 5, no. 2 (1980): 1–6.

Canino, Glorisa, and Margarita Alegria. "Understanding Psychopathology among the Adult and Child Latino Population from the United States and Puerto Rico: An Epidemiologic Perspective." In Villaruel et al., *Handbook of U.S. Latino Psychology: Developmental and Community-Based Perspectives,* 31–44.

Canino, Glorisa, Patrick E. Shrout, Maritza Rubio-Stipec, Hector R. Bird, Milagros Bravo, Rafael Ramirez, Ligia Chavez, Margarita Alegria, José J. Bauermeister, Ann Hohmann, Julio Ribera, Pedro Garcia, and Alfonso Martinez-Taboas. "The DSM-IV Rates of Child and Adolescent Disorders in Puerto Rico: Prevalence, Correlates, Service Use, and the Effects of Impairment." *Archives of General Psychiatry* 6, no. 1 (2004): 84–93.

Cantu, Norma Elia, and Olga Najera-Ramirez. *Chicana Traditions: Continuity and Change.* Urbana: University of Illinois Press, 2002.

Carballo-Dieguez, Alex. "Hispanic Culture, Gay Male Culture and AIDS: Counseling Implications." *Journal of Counseling and Development* 68, no. 1 (1989): 26–30.

Carlo, Gustavo, Francisco A. Villaruel, Margarita Azmitia, and Natasha J. Cabrera. "Perspectives and Recommendations for Future Directions in U.S. Latino

Psychology." In Villaruel et al., *Handbook of U.S. Latino Psychology: Developmental and Community-Based Perspectives,* 15–30. Thousand Oaks: Sage Publications, 2009.

Carrillo, Ricardo, and Jerry Tello, eds. *Family Violence and Men of Color: Healing the Wounded Male Spirit.* 2nd ed. New York: Springer, 2008.

Carrillo, Ricardo, and Maria Zarza. "Fire and Firewater: A Co-occurring Clinical Treatment Model for Domestic Violence, Substance Abuse, and Trauma. In *Family Violence and Men of Color: Healing the Wounded Male Spirit.* 2nd ed., ed. Ricardo Carrillo and Jerry Tello, 61–84. New York: Springer, 2008.

Casey Family Programs. *"Latino Children in Child Welfare"* (fact sheet), 2010. www.casey.org.

Cass, Vivienne. "Homosexual Identity Formation: A Theoretical Model." *Journal of Homosexuality* 4, no. 3 (1979): 219–35.

Castañeda, Donna. "The Close Relationship Context and HIV Risk Reduction Behavior among Latinas/os." *Sex Roles* 42 (2000): 551–80.

Castañeda, Xochitl. "Health Insurance Coverage in the United States." *California–Mexico Health Initiative Fact Sheet.* Berkeley: University of California Berkeley School of Public Health, 2005.

Castillo, Ana. *Massacre of the Dreamers: Essays on Xicanisma.* Albuquerque: University of New Mexico Press, 1995.

Castro, Felipe G. "A Cultural Approach for Promoting Resilience among Adjudicated Mexican American Youth. In *Race, Culture, Psychology and Law,* ed. Kimberly Holt Barrett and William H. George, 327–42. Thousand Oaks, CA: Sage Publications, 2005.

Cauce, Ana M., and Melanie Domenech Rodriguez. "Latino Families: Myths and Realities." In *Latino Children and Families in the United States: Current Research and Future Directions,* ed. Josefina M. Contreras, Kathryn A. Kearns, and Angela Neal Barnett, 3–26. Westport, CT: Praeger, 2002.

Centers for Disease Control and Prevention. *Depression among Women of Reproductive Age and Postpartum Depression: Factsheet.* Atlanta: Department of Health and Human Services, Centers for Disease Control and Prevention, 2010.

———. "HIV/AIDS among Hispanics/Latinos: Factsheet." Atlanta: Department of Health and Human Services, Centers for Disease Control and Prevention, 2005.

———. "HIV/AIDS among Women: Factsheet." Atlanta: Department of Health and Human Services, Centers for Disease Control and Prevention, 2008a.

———. "Prevalence of Autism Spectrum Disorders." Atlanta: Department of Health and Human Services, Centers for Disease Control and Prevention, 2008b.

Cervantes, Joseph M., Olga L. Mejia, and Amalia Guerrero Mena. "Serial Migration and the Assessment of Extreme and Unusual Hardship with Undocumented Latina/o Families." *Hispanic Journal of Behavioral Sciences* 32, no. 2 (2010): 275–91.

Cervantes, Richard C., and Maria Felix-Ortiz. "Substance Abuse among Chicanos and Other Mexican Groups." In *The Handbook of Chicana/o Psychology and Mental Health,* ed. Roberto Velazquez, Leticia Arellano, and Brian McNeill, 267–84. Mahwah, NJ: Lawrence Erlbaum, 2004.

Chabram-Dernersesian, Angie, and Adela de la Torre. *Speaking from the Body: Latinas on Health and Culture.* Tucson: University of Arizona Press, 2008.

Chamorro, Rebecca, and Yvette G. Flores-Ortiz. "Acculturation and Disordered Eating Patterns among Mexican American Women." *International Journal of Eating Disorders* 28, no. 1 (2000): 125–29. Reprinted in *Latina Health in the United States: A Public Health Reader,* ed. Marilyn Aguirre-Molina and Carlos W. Molina. San Francisco: Jossey-Bass, 2003.

Chávez, Denise. *Loving Pedro Infante: A Novel.* New York: Farrar, Straus and Giroux, 2001.

Chávez-García, Miroslava. *States of Delinquency: Race and Science in the Making of California's Juvenile Justice System.* Los Angeles and Berkeley: University of California Press, 2012.

Choi, Namkee G., and Jinseok Kim. "Age Group Differences in Depressive Symptoms among Older Adults with Functional Impairments." *Health and Social Work* 32, no. 3 (2007): 177–88.

Cisneros, Sandra. *The House on Mango Street.* New York: Random House, 1984.

Cook, Benjamin, Nicholas Carson, and Margarita Alegria. "Assessing Racial/Ethnic Differences in the Social Consequences of Early-Onset Psychiatric Disorder." *Journal of Health Care for the Poor and Underserved* 21, no. 2 (2010): 49–66.

Costello, E. Jane, Scott N. Compton, Gordon Keeler, and Adrian Angold. "Relationships between Poverty and Psychopathology: A Natural Experiment." *Journal of the American Medical Association* 290, no. 15 (2003): 2023–29.

Covington, Stephanie S. "Women and Addiction: A Trauma-Informed Approach." *Journal of Psychoactive Drugs,* SARC supplement 5, (2008): 377–85.

Davalos, Karen Mary. "La Quinceañera and the Keen-say-an-Yair-uh: The Politics of Making Gender and Ethnicity in Chicago." *Voces: A Journal of Chicana/Latina Studies* 1, no. 1 (1997): 57–68.

Deardorff, Juliana, Jeanne M. Tschann, and Elena Flores. "Sexual Values among Latino Youth: Measurement Development Using a Culturally Based Approach." *Culture Diversity and Ethnic Minority Psychology* 14, no. 2 (2008): 138–46.

de la Torre, Adela, and Antonio Estrada. *Mexican Americans and Health: ¡Sana! ¡Sana!* Tucson: University of Arizona Press, 2001.

de la Torre, Adela, Rosa Gomez-Camacho, and Alexis Alvarez. "Making the Case for Health Hardship: Examining the Mexican Health Care System in Cancellation of Removal Proceedings." *Georgetown Immigration Law Journal* 25, no. 1 (2010): 93–116.

Delgado, Jane. *Salud: A Latina's Guide to Total Health*. New York: Harper Collins, 2002.

Delgado-Gaitan, Concha. "*Consejos:* The Power of Cultural Narratives." *Anthropology and Education Quarterly* 25, no. 3 (1994): 298–316.

Diaz, Manuela, and Alicia Lieberman. "Use of Play in Child–Parent Psychotherapy with Preschoolers Traumatized by Domestic Violence." In *Play Therapy for Preschool Children,* ed. Charles E. Schaefer, 131–56. Washington, DC: American Psychological Association, 2010.

Diaz, Rafael M. *Latino Gay Men and AIDS: Culture, Sexuality and High-Risk Behavior*. New York: Routledge, 1998.

Diaz, Rafael M., and George Ayala. "Love, Passion and Rebellion: Ideologies of HIV Risk among Latino Gay Men in the USA." *Culture, Health and Sexuality* 1, no. 3 (1999): 277–93.

Diaz, Rafael M., Eduardo Morales, Edward Bein, Eugene Dilán, and Richard A. Rodriguez. "Predictors of Sexual Risk in Latino Gay/Bisexual Men: The Role of Demographic, Developmental, Social Cognitive, and Behavioral Variables." *Hispanic Journal of Behavioral Sciences* 21, no. 4 (1999): 480–501.

Diaz-Guerrero, Rogelio. *Psychology of the Mexican: Culture and Personality*. Austin: University of Texas Press, 1975.

Duran, Eduardo, and Bonnie Duran. *Native American Postcolonial Psychology*. Albany: State University of New York Press, 1995.

Echeverria, Sandra, and Ana Diez-Roux. "Emergent Chronic Conditions." In Aguirre-Molina, Borrell, and Vega, *Health Issues in Latino Males,* 158–82.

Eisenberg, Marla E., and Michael D. Resnick. "Suicidality among Gay, Lesbian and Bisexual Youth: The Role of Protective Factors." *Journal of Adolescent Health* 39, no. 5 (2006): 662–68.

Escobar, Javier, Jacqueline M. Golding, Richard L. Hough, Marvin Karno, M. Audrey Burnman, and Kenneth B. Wells. "Somatization in the Community: Relationship to Disability and Use of Services." *American Journal of Public Health* 77, no. 7 (1987): 837–40.

Espin, Oliva. "Cultural and Historical Influences on Sexuality in Hispanic/Latin Women: Implications for Therapy. In *Latina Realities: Essays on Healing, Migration and Sexuality,* ed. Oliva Espin, 83–96. Boulder, CO: Westview Press, 1987.

———. "Gender, Sexuality, Language, and Migration." In *Cultural Psychology of Immigrants,* ed. Ramaswami Mahalingam, 241–58. Mahwah, NJ: Lawrence Erlbaum, 2006.

———. " . . . An Illness We Catch from American Women? The Multiple Identities of Latina Lesbians." *Women and Therapy* 35, nos. 1–2 (2012): 45–56.

———. "Issues of Identity in the Psychology of Latina Lesbians. In *Latina Realities: Essays on Healing, Migration and Sexuality,* ed. Oliva Espin, 97–110. Boulder, CO: Westview Press, 1987.

———. *Women Crossing Boundaries: The Psychology of Immigration and the Transformations of Sexuality.* New York: Routledge, 1999.

Falicov, Celia. *Latino Families in Therapy: A Guide to Multicultural Practice.* New York: Guilford Press, 1998.

Finch, Brian K., Bohdan Kolody, and William A. Vega. "Perceived Discrimination and Depression among Mexican Origin Adults in California." *Journal of Health and Social Behavior* 41, no. 3 (2000): 295–313.

Flores, Consuelo, Diane Zelman, and Yvette Flores. "'I Have Not a Want but a Hunger to Feel No Pain': Mexican Immigrant Women with Chronic Pain: Narratives and Psychotherapeutic Implications." *Women and Therapy* 35, nos. 1–2 (2012): 31–44.

Flores, Elena, Jeanne M. Tschann, and Barbara VanOss Marin. "Latina Adolescents: Predicting Intentions to Have Sex." *Adolescence* 37, no. 148 (2002): 659–79.

Flores, Elena, Jeanne M. Tschann, Barbara VanOss Marin, and Philip Pantoja. "Marital Conflict and Acculturation among Mexican American Husbands and Wives." *Cultural Diversity and Ethnic Minority Psychology* 10, no. 1 (2004): 39–52.

Flores, Yvette G. "Embodying Dementia: Remembrances of Memory Loss." In *Speaking from the Body: Latinas on Health and Culture,* ed. Angie Chabram-Dernersesian and Adela de la Torre, 31–43. Tucson: University of Arizona Press, 2008.

———. "On Becoming an Elder: An Immigrant Latina Therapist Narrative." In *Women and Therapy in the Last Third of Life,* ed. Valory Mitchell, 13–28. New York: Routledge, 2010.

———. "Parenting." In *Encyclopedia Latina: History, Culture, and Society in the United States,* ed. Ilan Stavans, 316–22. Danbury, CT: Scholastic Library, 2005a.

———. "Rape." In *Latinas in the United States: An Historical Perspective,* ed. Virginia Sanchez Korrol, Vicki L. Ruiz, and Carlos Cruz, 611–13. Bloomington: Indiana University Press, 2005b.

———. "*La Salud*: Latina Adolescents Constructing Identities, Negotiating Health Decisions." In *Latina Girls: Voices of Adolescent Strength in the United States,* ed. Jill Denner and Bianca L. Guzmán, 199–211. New York: New York University Press, 2006.

Flores, Yvette, Ladson Hinton, Judith C. Barker, Carol E. Franz, and Alexandra Velasquez. "Beyond Familism: Ethics of Care of Latina Caregivers of Elderly Parents with Dementia." *Health Care for Women International* 30, no. 12 (2009): 1055–72.

Flores, Yvette, and Enriqueta Valdez Curiel. "Conflict Resolution and Intimate Partner Violence among Mexicans on Both Sides of the Border." In *Mexicans in California: Transformations and Challenges,* ed. Patricia Zavella and Ramón Gutiérrez, 183–216. Urbana: University of Illinois Press, 2009.

Flores, Yvette, Enriqueta Valdez Curiel, and Ana Fierro. "Intimate Partner Violence and Depressive Symptomatology among Rural Mexican Women." Unpublished manuscript, University of California, Davis, 2011.

Flores-Ortiz, Yvette G. "The Broken Covenant: Incest in Latino Families." *Voces: A Journal of Chicana/Latina Studies* 1, no. 1 (1997a): 48–70.

———. "Domestic Violence in Chicano Families." In *The Handbook of Chicana/o Psychology and Mental Health,* ed. Roberto Velazquez, Leticia Arellano, and Brian McNeill, 267–84. Mahwah, NJ: Lawrence Erlbaum, 2004.

———. "Fostering Accountability: A Reconstructive Dialogue with a Couple with a History of Violence." In *101 More Interventions in Family Therapy,* ed. Thorena Nelson and Terry Trepper, 389–96. New York: Haworth Press, 1998.

———. "Injustice in the Family." In *Family Therapy with Hispanics,* ed. Maria T. Flores and Gabrielle Carey, 251–93. Boston: Allyn and Bacon, 1999.

———. "Levels of Acculturation, Marital Satisfaction, and Depression among Chicana Workers: A Psychological Perspective." *Aztlan* 20, nos. 1 and 2 (1993a): 151–75.

———. "La Mujer y la Violencia: A Culturally Based Model for the Understanding and Treatment of Domestic Violence in Chicana/Latina Communities." In *Chicana Critical Issues,* ed. Norma Alarcón, 169–82. Berkeley: Third Woman Press, 1993b.

———. "Re/membering the Body: Latina Testimonies of Social and Family Violence." In *Violence and the Body: Race, Gender, and the State,* ed. Arturo J. Aldama, 347–59. Bloomington: Indiana University Press, 2003.

———. "The Role of Cultural and Gender Values in Alcohol Use Patterns among Chicana/Latina High School and University Students: Implications for AIDS Prevention." *International Journal of Addictions* 29, no. 9 (1994): 1149–71.

———. "Voices from the Couch: The Co-Construction of a Chicana Psychology." In *Living Chicana Theory,* ed. Carla Trujillo, 102–22. Berkeley: Third Woman Press, 1997b.

———. "Why Did He Want to Hurt Me? All I Ever Did Was Love Him: Understanding Sexual Violence in Latino Marriages." In *Transforming a Rape Culture*, 2nd ed., ed. Emily Buchwald, Pamela R. Fletcher, and Martha Roth, 129–38. Minneapolis: Milkweed Editions, 2005.

Flores-Ortiz, Yvette, Marcelo Esteban, and Ricardo Carrillo. "La violencia en la familia: Un modelo contextual de terapia intergeneracional." *Revista Interamericana de Psicología* 28, no. 2 (1994): 235–50.

Flores-Ortiz, Yvette, Enriqueta Valdez Curiel, and Patricia Andrade. "Intimate Partner Violence and Couple Interaction among Women from Mexico City and Jalisco." *Journal of Border Health* 7, no. 1 (2002): 33–42.

Franklin, Anderson J. *From Brotherhood to Manhood: How Black Men Rescue Their Relationships and Dreams from the Invisibility Syndrome.* New York: Wiley, 2004.

———. "Therapy with African American Men." *Families in Society: Journal of Contemporary Human Services* 73, no. 6 (1997): 350–55.

Franklin, Anderson J., and Nancy Boyd-Franklin. "Invisibility Syndrome: A Clinical Model of the Effects of Racism on African American Males." *American Journal of Orthopsychiatry* 70, no. 1 (2000): 33–41.

Freeman, Jennifer, Davis Epston, and Dean Lobovits. *Playful Approaches to Serious Problems*. New York: W. W. Norton, 1997.

Friedman, Samuel R., Hannah L. Cooper, Barbara Tempalski, M. Keem, Robert Friedman, Peter L. Flom, and Don C. Des Jarlais. "Relationships of Deterrence and Law Enforcement to Drug-Related Harms among Drug Injectors in US Metropolitan Areas." *AIDS* 20, no. 1 (2006): 93–99.

Fuentes, Carlos. *El espejo enterrado*. Madrid: Taurus, 1998.

Gallagher-Thompson, Dolores, Meagan C. Leary, Celine Ossinalde, and Josue J. Romero. "Hispanic Caregivers of Older Adults with Dementia: Cultural Issues in Outreach and Intervention." *Group* 21, no. 2 (1997): 211–32.

Gallegos-Castillo, Angela. "La Casa: Negotiating Family Cultural Practices, Constructing Identities." In *Latina Girls: Voices of Adolescent Strength in the United States,* ed. Jill Denner and Bianca L. Guzmán, 44–58. New York: New York University Press, 2006.

Gándara, Patricia. *Fragile Futures: Risk and Vulnerability among Latino High Achievers*. Policy Information Report. Princeton: ETS, 2005a.

———. *Latino Achievement: Identifying Models That Foster Success*. Storrs: National Center for the Gifted and Talented, University of Connecticut, 2005b.

Gándara, Patricia, Gary Orfield, and Catherine L. Horn, eds. *Expanding Opportunity in Higher Education: Leveraging Promise*. Albany: SUNY Press, 2006.

Gándara, Patricia, Russell Rumberger, Julie Maxwell-Jolly, and Rebecca Callahan. "English Learners in California Schools: Unequal Resources, Unequal Outcomes." *Education Policy Analysis Archives* 11, no. 36 (2003).

Garcia, Eugene E., and Danielle M. Gonzales. *Pre-K and Latinos: The Foundation for America's Future*. Washington, DC: Pre-K Now, 2006.

Gaspar de Alba, Alicia. "The Chicana/Latina Dyad, Or Identity and Perception." *Latino Studies* 1, no.1 (2003a): 106–14.

———. *Velvet Barrios: Popular Culture and Chicana/o Sexualities*. New York: Palgrave Macmillan, 2003b.

Gibson, Margaret, Patricia Gándara, and Jill Peterson Koyama, eds. *School Connections: U.S. Mexican Youth, Peers, and School Achievement*. New York: Teacher's College Press, 2004.

Gil, Andres, and William Vega. "Alcohol, Tobacco, and Other Drugs." In Aguirre-Molina, Borrell, and Vega, *Health Issues in Latino Males,* 99–122.

González, Hector M., Mary Haan, and Ladson Hinton. "Acculturation and the Prevalence of Depression in Older Mexican Americans: Baseline Results of the Sacramento Area Latino Study on Aging." *Journal of the American Geriatric Society* 49, no. 7 (2001): 948–53.

González, Hector M., Wassim Tarraf, Keith E. Whitfield, and William A. Vega. "The Epidemiology of Major Depression and Ethnicity in the United States." *Journal of Psychiatric Research* 44, no. 15 (2010): 1043–51.

Gonzalez, Nancy, Fairlee C. Fabrett, and George P. Knight. "Acculturation, Enculturation and the Psychosocial Adaptation of Latino Youth." In Aguirre-Molina,
Borrell, and Vega, *Health Issues in Latino Males,* 113–34.

Goodman, Catherine Chase, and Merril Silverstein. "Latina Grandmothers Raising
Grandchildren: Acculturation and Psychological Well-Being." *International Journal of Aging and Human Development* 60, no. 4 (2005): 305–16.

Gould, Madelyn S., Drew Velting, Marjorie Kleinman, Christopher Lucas, John Gra-
ham Thomas, and Michelle Chung. "Teenagers' Attitudes about Coping Strategies
and Help-Seeking Behavior for Suicidality." *Journal of the American Academy of
Child and Adolescent Psychiatry* 43, no. 9 (2004): 1124–33.

Grant, Bridget F., Frederick S. Stinson, Deborah S. Hasin, Deborah A. Dawson,
S. Patricia Chou, and Karyn Anderson. "Immigration and Lifetime Prevalence
of *DSM-IV* Psychiatric Disorders among Mexican Americans and Non-Hispanic
Whites in the United States: Results from the National Epidemiologic Survey on
Alcohol and Related Conditions." *Archives of General Psychiatry* 61, no. 12 (2004):
1226–33.

Grau, Josefina, Margarita Azmitia, and Justin Quattlebaum. "Latino Families, Parenting, Relational and Developmental Processes. In Villaruel et al., *Handbook of
U.S. Latino Psychology: Developmental and Community-Based Perspectives,* 153–70.

Guarnaccia, Peter J., Jacqueline Lowe Angel, and Ronald Angel. "The Impacts of
Farm Work on Health: Analyses of the Hispanic Health and Nutrition Examination Survey." *International Migration Review* 26, no. 1 (1992): 111–32.

Guarnaccia, Peter J., Roberto Lewis-Fernandez, Igda Martinez Pincay, Patrick
Shrout, Jing Guo, Maria Torres, Glorisa Canino, and Margarita Alegria. "*Ataque
de nervios* as a Marker of Social and Psychiatric Vulnerability: Results from the
NLAAS." *International Journal of Social Psychiatry* 56, no. 3 (2010): 298–309.

Gurin, Patricia, and Betty Mae Morrison. *Two-Way Socialization Processes in the Classroom. Final Report.* Unpublished research report, 1980.

Haan, Mary M., Dan M. Mungas, Hector M. Gonzalez, Teresa A. Ortiz, Ananth
Acharya, and William J. Jagust. "Prevalence of Dementia in Older Latinos: The
Influence of Type 2 Diabetes Mellitus, Stroke and Genetic Factors." *Journal of the
American Geriatric Society* 51, no. 2 (2003): 169–77.

Hardy, Kenneth V., and Tracey A. Laszloffy. *Teens Who Hurt: Clinical Interventions to
Break the Cycle of Adolescent Violence.* New York: Guilford Press, 2005.

Hayes-Bautista, David E. *Nueva California.* Berkeley: University of California Press,
2004.

Hayes-Bautista, David E., and Jorge Chapa. *Burden of Support: Young Latinos in an
Aging Society.* Stanford: Stanford University Press, 1990.

Hayes-Bautista, David E., Werner O. Schink, and Jorge Chapa. *The Health of Latino
California: Chartbook.* Los Angeles: Center for the Study of Latino Health, Division

of General Internal Medicine and Health Services Research, Dept. of Medicare, School of Medicine, UCLA, 1998.

Herman, Judith Lewis. *Trauma and Recovery*. New York: Basic Books, 1992.

Hing, Bill Ong. *Defining America through Immigration Policy*. Philadelphia: Temple University Press, 2004.

Hinton, Ladson, Ester C. Apesoa-Varano, Hector M. González, Sergio Aguilar-Gaxiola, Judith C. Barker, Megan Dwight-Johnson, Cindi Tran, Ramiro Zuniga, and Jürgen Unutzer. "Falling through the Cracks: Gaps in Depression Care for Older Mexican-Origin and White Men." *International Journal of Geriatric Psychiatry*. In press.

Hinton, Ladson, Darren Chambers, and Alexandra Velasquez. "Making Sense of Behavioral Disturbances in Persons with Dementia: Latino Family Caregiver Attributions of Neuropsychiatric Inventory Domains." *Alzheimer Disease and Associated Disorders* 23, no. 4 2009: 401–5.

Hinton, Ladson, Yvette Flores, Carol Franz, Isabel Hernandez, and Linda S. Mitteness. "The Borderlands of Primary Care: Physician and Family Perspectives on 'Troublesome Behaviors' of People with Dementia." In *Thinking about Dementia: Culture, Loss, and the Anthropology of Senility,* ed. Annette Leibing and Lawrence Cohen, 43–63. New Brunswick, NJ: Rutgers University Press, 2006.

Hinton, Ladson, Carol E. Franz, Getha Reddy, Yvette Flores, Richard L. Kravitz, and Judith C. Barker. "Practice Constraints, Behavioral Problems, and Dementia Care: Primary Care Physicians' Perspectives." *Journal of General Internal Medicine* 22, no. 1 (2007): 1–6.

Hinton, Ladson, Yolanda Hagar, Nancy West, Hector M. González, Dan Mungas, Laurel Beckett, and Mary N. Haan. "Longitudinal Influences of Partner Depression on Cognitive Functioning in Latino Spousal Pairs." *Dementia and Geriatric Cognitive Disorders* 27, no. 6 (2009): 491–500.

Hinton, Ladson, Sarah Tomaszewski Farias, and Jacob Wegelin. "Neuropsychiatric symptoms Are Associated with Disability in Cognitively Impaired Latino Elderly with and without Dementia: Results from the Sacramento Area Latino Study on Aging." *International Journal of Geriatric Psychiatry* 23, no. 1 (2008): 102–8.

Homan, Russell, Patricia Homan, and Olveen Carrasquillo. "Health Coverage, Utilization and Expenditures among Latino Men." In Aguirre-Molina, Borrell, and Vega, *Health Issues in Latino Males,* 229–48.

Hurtado, Aida. *Voicing Chicana Feminisms: Young Women Speak Out on Sexuality and Identity*. New York: New York University Press, 2003.

Hurtado, Aida, and Patricia Gurin. *Chicana/o Identity in a Changing U.S. Society: ¿Quien Soy? ¿Quiénes Somos?* Tucson: University of Arizona Press, 2004.

Institute on Women and Criminal Justice. Quick Facts: Women & Criminal Justice— 2009. Women's Prison Association, 2009. http://www.wpaonline.org/.

Johnson, Michael P. *A Typology of Domestic Violence: Intimate Terrorism, Violent Resistance, and Situational Couple Violence.* Lebanon, NH: Northeastern University Press and University Press of New England, 2008.

Johnson, Michael P., and Janel M. Leone. "The Differential Effects of Intimate Terrorism and Situational Couple Violence." *Journal of Family Issues* 26, no. 3 (2005): 322–49.

Keough, Meghan E., Kiara R. Timpano, and Norman B. Schmidt. "*Ataques de Nervios*: Culturally Bound and Distinct from Panic Attacks?" *Depression and Anxiety* 26, no. 1 (2009): 16–21.

Kessler, Ronald C., and Kathleen R. Merikangas. "Lifetime Prevalence and Age-of-Onset Distributions of *DSM-IV* Disorders in the National Comorbidity Survey Replication." *Archives of General Psychiatry* 62 no. 6 (2005): 593–602.

Kleinman, Arthur. *The Illness Narratives: Suffering, Healing and the Human Condition.* New York: Basic Books, 1988.

Koss-Chioino, Joan D., and Luis A. Vargas. *Working with Latino Youth: Culture, Development and Context.* San Francisco: Jossey-Bass, 1999.

Lewis-Fernandez, Roberto, Pedro Garrido-Castillo, Mari Bennasar Carmen, Elsie M. Parrilla, Amaro J. Laria, Guoguang Ma, and Eva Petkova. "Dissociation, Childhood Trauma and *Ataque de Nervios* among Puerto Rican Psychiatric Outpatients." *American Journal of Psychiatry* 159 (2002): 1603–5.

Lipsky, Sherry, and Raul Caetano. "Impact of Intimate Partner Violence on Unmet Need for Mental Health Care: Results from the NSDUH." *Psychiatric Services: A Journal of the American Psychiatric Association* 58, no. 6 (2007): 822–29.

Lipsky, Sherry, and Raul Caetano. "The Role of Race/Ethnicity in the Relationship between Emergency Department Use and Intimate Partner Violence: Findings from the 2002 National Survey on Drug Use and Health." *American Journal of Public Health* 97, no. 12 (2007): 2246–52.

Lipsky, Sherry, Raul Caetano, Craig Field, and Shahrzad Bazargan. "Violence-Related Injury and Intimate Partner Violence in an Urban Emergency Department." *Journal of Trauma* 5, no. 2 (2004): 352.

Lipsky, Sherry, Raul Caetano, Craig A. Field, and Gregory L. Larkin. "The Role of Intimate Partner Violence, Race, and Ethnicity in Help-Seeking Behaviors." *Ethnicity and Health* 11, no. 1 (2006): 81–100.

Lopez, Steven Regeser, and Peter J. Guarnaccia. "Cultural Psychopathology: Uncovering the Social World of Mental Illness." *Annual Review of Psychology* 51 (2000): 571–98.

Lopez, Steven R., Jorge I. Ramirez Garcia, Jodie B. Ullman, Alex Kopelowicz, Janis Jenkins, Nicholas J. K. Breitborde, and Perla Placencia. "Cultural Variability in the Manifestation of Expressed Emotion." *Family Process* 48, no. 2 (2009): 179–94.

Lopez-Rangel, Elena. "Latino Culture." In *Cultural and Ethnic Diversity: A Guide for Genetics Professionals,* ed. Nancy L. Fisher, 19–35. Baltimore: Johns Hopkins University Press, 1996.

Lown, E. Anne, and William A. Vega. "Prevalence and Predictors of Emotional and Physical Abuse among Mexican American Women: The Role of Acculturation." *American Journal of Public Health* 91, no. 3 (2001): 441–45.

Madanes, Cloé. *Sex, Love, and Violence: Strategies for Transformation*. New York: Norton, 1990.

Madanes, Cloé, James P. Keim, and Dinah Smelser. *Violencia masculina*. Barcelona: Granica, 1997.

Massachusetts Department of Elementary and Secondary Education. *Nutrition, Health and Safety: Youth Risk Behavior Survey*. 2007. http://www.doe.mass.edu/cnp/programs/yrbs.

McCubbin, Laurie, and Anthony Marsella. "Native Hawaiians and Psychology: The Cultural and Historical Context of Indigenous Ways of Knowing." *Cultural Diversity and Ethnic Minority Psychology* 15, no. 4 (2009): 374–87.

Mennen, F. Elizabeth. "Sexual Abuse in Latina Girls: Their Functioning and Comparison with White and African American Girls." *Hispanic Journal of Behavioral Sciences* 16, no. 4 (1994): 475–86.

Minuchin, Salvador, Braulio Montalvo, Bernard Guerney, Bernice Rossman, and Florence Schumer. *Families of the Slums: An Exploration of Their Structure and Treatment*. New York: Basic Books, 1967.

Miranda, Jeanne, Juned Siddique, Claudia Der-Martirosian, and Thomas R. Belin. "Depression among Latina Immigrant Mothers Separated from Their Children." *Psychiatric Services* 56, no. 6 (2005): 717–20.

Mora, Juana. "The Treatment of Alcohol Dependency among Latinas: A Feminist, Cultural, and Community Perspective." In *Latina Health in the U.S.: A Public Health Reader,* ed. Marilyn Aguirre-Molina and Carlos W. Molina, 272–84. San Francisco: Jossey-Bass, 2003.

Moraga, Cherrie, and Gloria Anzaldúa. *This Bridge Called My Back: Writings by Radical Women of Color*. New York: Kitchen Table/ Women of Color Press, 1983.

Morales, Eduardo S. "Ethnic Minority Families and Minority Gays and Lesbians." In *Homosexuality and Family Relations,* ed. Frederick W. Bozett and Marvin D. Sussman, 272–97. New York: Haworth Press, 1990.

Muñoz, Ricardo F., Pim Cuijpers, Filip Smit, Alinne Z. Barrera, and Yan Leykin. "Prevention of Major Depression." *Annual Review of Clinical Psychology* 6 (2010): 181–212. www.ncbi.nlm.nih.gov/pubmed/20192789.

Mustanski, Brian S., Robert Garofalo, and Erin M. Emerson. "Mental Health Disorders, Psychological Distress, and Suicidality in a Diverse Sample of Lesbian, Gay, Bisexual, and Transgender Youths." *American Journal of Public Health* 100, no. 12 (2010): 2426–32.

National Center for Health Statistics. *Health, United States, 2011: With Special Feature on Socioeconomic Status and Health*. Hyattsville, MD: National Center for Health Statistics, 2012.

National Institute of Mental Health. *Mood Disorders Fact Sheet*. October 2005. http://www.nimh.nih.gov.

Nemoto, Tooru, Don Operario, and JoAnne Keatley. "Health and Social Services for Male-to-Female Transgender Persons of Color in San Francisco." *International Journal of Transgenderism* 8, nos. 2–3 (2005): 5–19.

Nemoto, Tooru, Don Operario, JoAnne Keatley, Lei Han, and Toho Soma. "HIV Risk Behaviors among Male-to-Female Transgender Persons of Color in San Francisco." *American Journal of Public Health* 94, no. 7 (2004): 1193–99.

Newton, Frank. "The Mexican American Emic System of Mental Health: An Exploratory Study." In *Family and Mental Health in the Mexican American Community*, ed. Juan Manuel Casas and Susan E. Keefe, 69–90. Los Angeles: UCLA Spanish Speaking Mental Health Research Center, 1978.

Novak, Kate, and Judith Riggs. *Hispanics/Latinos and Alzheimer's Disease*. [La enfermedad de Alzheimer entre la población hispana/latina.] Chicago: Alzheimer's Association, 2004.

Ogbu, John U. *Minority Education and Caste: The American System in Cross-Cultural Perspective*. San Diego: Academic Press, 1978.

Organista, Kurt. *Solving Latino Psychosocial and Health Problems: Theory, Research and Populations*. Hoboken, NJ: John Wiley and Sons, 2007.

Ortegon, Martha, and Deborah Werner. "Resources for Latina Population, California Women Children and Families TA Project: A Project of Children and Family Futures." Funded by the California Dept. of Alcohol and Drug Programs. 2008.

Paz, Octavio. *The Labyrinth of Solitude: Life and Thought in Mexico*. New York: Grove Press, 1962.

Perez, Emma. "Borderland Queers: The Challenges of Excavating the Invisible and Unheard." *Frontiers: A Journal of Women's Studies* 24, nos. 2–3 (2003): 122–31.

Perilla, Julia, Roger Bakeman, and Fran H. Norris. "Culture and Domestic Violence: The Ecology of Abused Latinas." *Violence and Victims* 9, no. 4 (1994): 325–39.

Perilla, Julia L., Caroline A. Lippy, Alvina Rosales, and Josephine Vazquez Serrata. "Domestic Violence Prevalence: Philosophical, Methodological, and Cultural Considerations." In *Violence against Women and Children: Consensus, Critical Analyses, and Emergent Priorities*. Vol. 1, *Mapping the Terrain*. Washington, DC: APA. In press.

Perilla, Julia L., Josephine Vazquez Serrata, Joanna Weinberg, and Caroline A. Lippy. "Integrating Women's Voices and Theory: A Comprehensive Domestic Violence Intervention for Latinas." *Women and Therapy* 35, nos. 1–2 (2012): 93–105.

Poe-Yamagata, Eileen, and M. A. Jones. *And Justice for Some: Differential Treatment of Minority Youth in the Justice System*. Washington: Youth Law Center, 2000.

Poe-Yamagata, Eileen, and Madeline Wardes Noya. "Race Disparities in the Juvenile Justice System." In *Race, Culture, Psychology and Law*, ed. Kimberly Holt Barrett and William H. George, 311–45. Thousand Oaks, CA: Sage, 2005.

Polo, Antonio, and Margarita Alegria. "Psychiatric Disorders and Mental Health Service Use among Latino Men in the United States." In Aguirre-Molina, Borrell, and Vega, *Health Issues in Latino Males,* 183–211.

Polo, Antonio J., and Steven Lopez. "Culture, Context, and the Internalizing Distress of Mexican American Youth." *Journal of Clinical Child and Adolescent Psychology* 38, no. 2 (2009): 1–13.

Portes, Alejandro, Patricia Fernandez-Kelly, and William Haller. "Segmented Assimilation on the Ground: The New Second Generation in Early Adulthood." *Ethnic and Racial Studies* 28, no. 6 (2005): 1000–1040.

Portes, Alejandro, and Min Zhou. "The New Second Generation: Segmented Assimilation and Its Variants among Post-1965 Immigrant Youth." *The Annals of the American Academy of Political and Social Sciences* 530, no. 1 (1993): 74–95.

Priel, Beatriz, and Avi Besser. "Perceptions of Early Relationships during the Transition to Motherhood: The Mediating Role of Social Support." *Infant Mental Health Journal* 23, no. 4 (2002): 343–60.

Quintana, Stephen M., and Nicholas C. Scull. "Latino Ethnic Identity." In Villaruel et al., *Handbook of U.S. Latino Psychology: Developmental and Community-Based Perspectives,* 81–98.

Quintana, Stephen M., and Elizabeth Vera. "Mexican-American Children's Representations of Ethnic Prejudice." *Hispanic Journal of Behavioral Sciences* 21, no. 4 (1999): 387–404.

Ramirez, Manuel III. *Multiracial/Multicultural Psychology: Mestizo Perspectives in Personality and Mental Health.* Lanham, MD: Rowman and Littlefield, 1998.

Ramos Lira, Luciana, Mary P. Koss, and Nancy Felipe Russo. "Mexican American Women's Definitions of Rape and Sexual Abuse." *Hispanic Journal of Behavioral Sciences* 21, no. 3 (1999): 236–65.

Ramos Lira, Luciana, Maria Teresa Saltijeral, and Gabriela Saldivar. "El miedo a la victimización y su relación con los medios de comunicación." *Salud Mental* 18, no. 2 (1995): 35–43.

Rios-Ellis, Britt. "Critical Disparities in Latino Mental Health: Transforming Research into Action." *National Council of La Raza* (2005): 6.

Rios-Ellis, Britt, Noelle Hurd, Antonio Duran, and Rocio A. Leon. *BE SAFE: A Cultural Competency Model for Latinos.* Washington, DC: National Minority AIDS Education and Training Center, 2005.

Rodriguez, Michael, Heidy Bauer, Yvette Flores-Ortiz, and Seline Skupinski-Quiroga. "Factors Affecting Patient–Physician Communication for Abused Latina and Asian Immigrant Women." *Journal of Family Practice* 47, no. 2 (1998): 309–11.

Rodriguez, Michael A., MarySue V. Heilemann, Eve Fielder, Alfonso Ang, Faustina Nevarez, and Carol M. Mangione. "Intimate Partner Violence, Depression, and PTSD among Pregnant Latina Women." *Annals of Family Medicine* 6, no. 1 (2008): 44–52.

Rodriguez, Michael A., Jeannette M. Valentine, John B. Son, and Marjani Muhammad. "Intimate Partner Violence and Barriers to Mental Health Care for Ethnically Diverse Populations of Women." *Trauma, Violence and Abuse* 10, no. 4 (2009): 358–74.

Rodriguez, Richard. "Psychotherapy with Gay Chicanos." In *The Handbook of Chicano Psychology and Mental Health,* ed. Robert Velasquez, Leticia M. Arellano, and Brian McNeil, 193–214. Mahwah, NJ: Lawrence Erlbaum, 2004.

Rumbaut, Ruben G. "The Crucible Within: Ethnic Identity, Self-Esteem, and Segmented Assimilation among Children of Immigrants." *International Immigration Review* 28, no. 4 (1994): 748–94.

Russo, Nancy F., and Jean E. Denious. "Violence in the Lives of Women Having Abortions: Implications for Public Policy and Practice." *Professional Psychology: Research and Practice* 32, no. 2 (2001): 142–50.

Salgado de Snyder, V. Nelly, Ma. de Jesus Diaz-Perez, and Victoria D. Ojeda. "The Prevalence of Nervios and Associated Symptomatology Among Inhabitants of Mexican Rural Communities." *Culture, Medicine and Psychiatry* 24, no. 4 (2000): 453–70.

Shetgiri, Rashmi, Sheryl Kataoka, Ninez A. Ponce, Glenn Flores, and Paul J. Chung. "Adolescent Fighting: Racial/Ethnic Disparities and the Importance of Families and Schools." *Academic Pediatrics* 10, no. 5 (2010): 323–29.

Siegel, Daniel J. *The Developing Mind: Second Edition: How Relationships and the Brain Interact to Shape Who We Are.* New York: Guilford Press, 2012.

Sluzki, Carlos E. "The 'Latin Lover' Revisited: An Ethnological–Communicational Analysis." In *Ethnicity and Family Therapy,* ed. Monica McGoldrick, John K. Pearce, and Joseph Giordano, 492–98. New York: Guilford, 1976.

Souza, Caridad. "Esta risa no es de loca." In the Latina Feminist Group, *Telling to Live: Latina Feminist Testimonios,* 114–22. Durham, NC: Duke University Press, 2001.

State of Hispanic Girls. Washington, DC: National Coalition of Hispanic Health and Human Service Organizations, 1999.

Stebleton, Michael J., Ronald L. Huesman, and Aliya Kuzhebekova. *"Do I Belong Here? Exploring Immigrant College Student Responses on the SERU Survey Sense of Belonging/Satisfaction Factor.* Occasional Research Paper. Berkeley: University of California Center for Studies in Higher Education, 2010.

Stein, Judith A., Marion Riedel, and Mary Jane Rotheram-Borus. "Parentification and Its Impact on Adolescent Children of Parents with AIDS." *Family Process* 38, no. 2 (1999): 193–208.

Steiner, V., and D. Paige. *Closing the Mental Health Gap: Eliminating Disparities in Treatment for Latinos.* Kansas City, MO: Mattie Rhodes Center, 2003.

Sue, Derald Wing. *Microaggressions in Everyday Life: Race, Gender, and Sexual Orientation.* New York: John Wiley and Sons, 2010.

Sue, Derald Wing, Cristina M. Capodilupo, Gina C. Torino, Jennifer M. Bucceri, Aisha M. B. Holder, Kevin L. Nadal, and Marta Esquilin. "Racial Microaggressions in Everyday Life: Implications for Clinical Practice." *American Psychologist* 62, no. 4 (2007): 271–86.

Szapocznik, Jose, David Santiesteban, Arturo T. Rio, Angel Perez-Vidal, William M. Kurtines. "Family Effectiveness Training to Prevent Behavioral Problems in Hispanic Adolescents." *Hispanic Journal of Behavioral Sciences* 11, no. 1 (1989): 4–27.

Tello, Jerry. "El Hombre Noble Buscando Balance: The Noble Man Searching for Balance." In *Family Violence and Men of Color: Healing the Wounded Male Spirit,* 2nd ed., ed. Ricardo Carrillo and Jerry Tello, 37–60. New York: Springer, 2008.

Tello, Jerry. *Cara y Corazón, Face and Heart: A Family Strengthening, Rebalancing, and Community Mobilization Process.* San Antonio: National Latino Children's Institute, 1994.

Tello, Jerry, Rebecca Mariá Barrera, Santiago Espinosa, and Maria Elena Riojas Lester. *Cara y Corazón = Face And Heart : A Family Strengthening Program for Those Who Have Experienced the Pain of Alcohol and Drug Dependent Homes.* Austin: Corporate Child Development Fund for Texas, 1991.

Torres, Lucas. "Predicting Levels of Latino Depression: Acculturation, Acculturative Stress, and Coping." *Cultural Diversity and Ethnic Minority Psychology* 16, no. 2 (2010): 256–63.

Trujillo, Carla, ed. *Chicana Lesbians: The Girls Our Mothers Warned Us About.* Berkeley: Third Woman Press, 2001.

———. "Sexual Identity and the Discontent of Differences." In *Ethnic and Cultural Diversity among Lesbians and Gay Men,* ed. Beverly Greene, 266–78. Thousand Oaks, CA: Sage Publications, 1997.

Turner, R. Jay, and Andres Gil. "Psychiatric and Substance Use Disorders in South Florida: Racial/Ethnic and Gender Contrasts in a Young Adult Cohort." *Archives of General Psychiatry* 59, no. 1 (2002): 43–50.

Umaña-Taylor, Adriana J., and Edna C. Alfaro. "Acculturative Stress and Adaptation." In Villaruel et al., *Handbook of U.S. Latino Psychology: Developmental and Community-Based Perspectives,* 15–152.

US Census Bureau. Quick Facts, 2008. http://quickfacts.census.gov/qfd/states/00000.html

———. Census Briefs, "Population Distribution and Change: 2000 to 2010, An Overview: Race and Hispanic Origin and the 2010 Census. Washington, DC: Department of the Census, 2011.

US Department of Health and Human Services. *Mental Health: Culture, Race and Ethnicity—A Supplement to Mental Health: A Report of the Surgeon General. Executive Summary.* Rockville, MD: US Department of Health and Human Services, Substance Abuse and Mental Health Services Administration, Center for Mental Health Services, 2001.

US Department of Health and Human Services, SAMHSA, Substance Abuse and Mental Health Services Administration. Newsroom, "National Survey Report." 2009. http://www.samhsa.gov/newsroom/advisories/1009152021.aspx.

US Department of Justice, Office of Juvenile Justice and Delinquency Prevention. Charles Puzzanchera, "Juvenile Arrests 2007." Washington, DC: Federal Bureau of Investigation, 2008.

van der Kolk, Bessel A. "The Body Keeps the Score: Memory and the Evolving Psychobiology of Post Traumatic Stress." *Harvard Review of Psychiatry* 1, no. 5 (1994): 253–65.

———. "Developmental Trauma Disorder." *Psychiatric Annals* 35, no. 5 (2005): 401–9.

———. "The Psychobiology of Posttraumatic Stress Disorder." *Journal of Clinical Psychiatry* 58, no. 9 (1997): 16–24.

Vega, William A., and Hortencia Amaro. "Good Health: Uncertain Prognosis." *Annual Review of Public Health* 14 (1994): 39–67.

Vega, William, Luisa N. Borrell, and Marilyn Aguirre-Molina. "Conclusions: New Directions for Research, Policy, and Programs Addressing the Health of Latino Males." In Aguirre-Molina, Borrell, and Vega, *Health Issues in Latino Males,* 261–67.

Vega, William A., Bohdan Kolody, and Sergio A. Aguilar-Gaxiola. Help-Seeking for Mental Health Problems among Mexican-Americans. *Journal of Immigrant Health* 3, no. 3 (2001): 133–40.

Vega, William A., Bohdan Kolody, Sergio A. Aguilar-Gaxiola, and Ralph Catalano. "Gaps in Service Utilization by Mexican Americans with Mental Health Problems." *American Journal of Psychiatry* 156, no. 6 (1999): 928–34.

Vega, William A., Bohdan Kolody, Sergio A. Aguilar-Gaxiola, Ethel Alderete, Ralph Catalano, and Jorge Caraveo-Anduaga. "Lifetime Prevalence of *DSM-III-R* Psychiatric Disorders among Urban and Rural Mexican Americans in California." *Archives of General Psychiatry* 55, no. 9 (1998): 771–78.

Velasquez, Roberto J., and Patricia Burton. "The Psychotherapy of Chicano Men." In Villaruel et al., *Handbook of U.S. Latino Psychology: Developmental and Community-Based Perspectives,* 177–92.

Vigil, Luis Diego. *A Rainbow of Gangs: Street Cultures in the Mega-City*. Austin: University of Texas Press, 2002.

Villa, Velentine V., Nancy Harada, and Anh-Luu Huynh-Hohnbaum. "The Causes and Consequences of Poor Health among Latino Vietnam Veterans: Parallels for Latino Veterans of the War in Iraq." In Aguirre-Molina, Borrell, and Vega, *Health Issues in Latino Males,* 123–38.

Villaruel, Francisco, Gustavo Carlo, Josefina Grau, Margarita Azmitia, Natasha J. Cabrera, and Jamie T. Chahin, eds. *Handbook of U.S. Latino Psychology: Developmental and Community-Based Perspectives*. Thousand Oaks, CA: Sage Publications, 2009.

Williams, David R. "The Health of U.S. Racial and Ethnic Populations." *Journals of Gerontology Series B* 60, special issue no. 2 (2005): 53–62.

Williams, David R., and Chiquita Collins. "U.S. Socioeconomic and Racial Differences in Health: Patterns and Explanations." *Annual Review of Sociology* 21 (1995): 349–86.

Williams, David R., and Pamela Braboy Jackson. "Social Sources of Racial Disparities in Health." *Health Affairs* 24, no. 2 (2005): 325–34.

Williams, David R., and Selina A. Mohammed. "Discrimination and Racial Disparities in Health: Evidence and Needed Research." *Journal of Behavioral Medicine* 32, no. 1 (2009): 20–47.

Williams, Norma. *The Mexican American Family: Tradition and Change*. Dix Hills, NY: General Hall, 1990.

Woodward, George. "Autism and Parkinson's Disease." *Medical Hypotheses* 56, no. 2 (2001): 246–49.

Ybarra, Lea. *Vietnam Veteranos: Chicanos Recall the War*. Austin: University of Texas Press, 2004.

Youth Risk Behavior Surveillance System (YRBSS). *Morbidity and Mortality Weekly Report* 5, no. 5 (2005): 1–108.

Zavella, Patricia. "Playing with Fire: The Gendered Construction of Chicana/Mexicana Sexuality." In *Gender/Sexuality Reader: Culture, History, Political Economy*, ed. Roger N. Lancester and Micaela di Leonardo, 392–408. New York: Routledge, 1997.

———. "Talking Sex: Chicanas and Mexicanas Theorize about Silences and Sexual Pleasures." In *Chicana Feminisms: A Critical Reader,* ed. Gabriela F. Arredondo, Aida Hurtado, Norma Klahn, Olga Najera-Ramirez, and Patricia Zavella, 228–53. Durham: Duke University Press, 2003.

Ziegler, Dave. *Traumatic Experience and the Brain*. Phoenix: Acacia, 2002.

■ INDEX

school, 8, 29–30

segmented assimilation, 7–8, 9

sexual abuse, 53, 62–66; childhood, 27–28; intimate partner violence, 64–66, 84–85; rape, incest, 64–65

sexuality, 12, 53–54, 100–118; AIDS, 101, 111; coming-of-age rituals, 102; gays and lesbians, 108–112; gender roles, 41–42; male, 105–107; sexual violence, 115–118; teen pregnancy, 101, 107–108. *See also* LGBT

substance abuse disorders, 68–73; addiction, 69, 70–72; mood disorders, 72; negative consequences, 73; primary substances abused, 68; risk factors, 68–69; substance intoxication, 71–72; withdrawal, 70–71

suicide, 41, 44, 55

Tello, Jerry: *cargas y regales* (gifts and burdens), 17; formulation of Chicano identity, 78–79

teen pregnancy, 101, 107–108

trauma, 54, 63, 65; anxiety, 21–23; historical, 1–3, 6, 8–9, 76, 105; intergenerational, 3–4, 16, 46, 54, 55; intimate partner violence, 84–85; parents' history, 17; symptoms, 62–64; war veterans, 89. *See also* PTSD (posttraumatic stress disorder)

◼ ABOUT THE AUTHOR

Born in Colon, Panama, and raised in San Jose, Costa Rica, and South Central Los Angeles, Yvette Flores learned early the impact of migration on individuals and families. Dr. Flores pursued undergraduate studies in psychology at UC Santa Barbara and a master's degree in Community-Clinical Psychology at CSU Long Beach, obtaining her doctorate in Clinical Psychology at UC Berkeley in 1982. Her life work has bridged psychology and Chicano studies and has focused on the physical and emotional well-being of immigrants and their US-born children. Her recent research and publications address the prevalence of intimate partner violence (IPV) among Mexican nationals and Mexicans in the United States, the relationship between depression and IPV in rural Mexican women, and caregiving patterns of spouses and adult children of elderly with dementia.

At present, Dr. Flores is part of a research team focusing on obesity prevention and healthy lifestyle promotion among Mexican-origin children and adults in Central California. Professor Flores is also part of several collaborative, binational research teams. A Fulbright fellow (Panama 1994) and a Fogarty Fellow (Mexico 1999), she has taught in Panama City and Costa Rica; she has also supervised doctoral and master's thesis students at the Universidad Nacional Autonóma de Mexico (UNAM), Universidad de Guadalajara, Centro Universitario Sur, and the Universidad de Costa Rica. Dr. Flores is an international consultant and trainer in the areas of illness prevention, program development, and cultural competency. She has maintained a private practice since 1986.

Chicana and Chicano Mental Health is a volume in the series *The Mexican American Experience,* a cluster of modular texts designed to provide greater flexibility in undergraduate education. Each book deals with a single topic concerning the Mexican American population. Instructors can create a semester-length course from any combination of volumes or may choose to use one or two volumes to complement other texts.

Additional volumes deal with the following subjects:

Mexican Americans and Health
Adela de la Torre and Antonio Estrada

Chicano Popular Culture
Charles M. Tatum

Mexican Americans and the US Economy
Arturo González

Mexican Americans and the Law
Reynaldo Anaya Valencia, Sonia R. García, Henry Flores, and José Roberto Juárez Jr.

Chicana/o Identity in a Changing US Society
Aída Hurtado and Patricia Gurin

Mexican Americans and the Environment
Devon G. Peña

Mexican Americans and the Politics of Diversity
Lisa Magaña

Mexican Americans and Language
Glenn A. Martínez

Chicano and Chicana Literature
Charles M. Tatum

Chicana and Chicano Art
Carlos Francisco Jackson

Immigration Law and the US–Mexico Border
Kevin R. Johnson and Bernard Trujillo

For more information, please visit
www.uapress.arizona.edu/textbooks/latino.htm